A Comprehensive Overview of HIV Infection

A Comprehensive Overview of HIV Infection

Edited by **Chris Stinson**

FOSTER
ACADEMICS

New Jersey

Published by Foster Academics,
61 Van Reypen Street,
Jersey City, NJ 07306, USA
www.fosteracademics.com

A Comprehensive Overview of HIV Infection
Edited by Chris Stinson

International Standard Book Number: 978-1-63242-011-4 (Hardback)

Printed in the United States of America.

Contents

            Mental Distress   **146**
            Peter J. Chipimo and Knut Fylkesnes

Chapter 9   **Persistence of HIV-Associated Neurocognitive Disorders in the**
            Era of Antiretroviral Therapy   **157**
            Jennifer M. King, Brigid K. Jensen, Patrick J. Gannon and Cagla Akay

            Permissions

            List of Contributors

Preface

This book has been an outcome of determined endeavour from a group of educationists in the field. The primary objective was to involve a broad spectrum of professionals from diverse cultural background involved in the field for developing new researches. The book not only targets students but also scholars pursuing higher research for further enhancement of the theoretical and practical applications of the subject.

A descriptive analysis of HIV and AIDS has been presented in this all-inclusive book. Along with the basic concepts of pathology, immunopathology and immunity, diagnosis and epidemiology to present-day clinical recommendations in management of AIDS/HIV including NeuroAIDS is discussed in detail. This book is an invaluable source of reference for those interested in the research and treatment of HIV infection.

It was an honour to edit such a profound book and also a challenging task to compile and examine all the relevant data for accuracy and originality. I wish to acknowledge the efforts of the contributors for submitting such brilliant and diverse chapters in the field and for endlessly working for the completion of the book. Last, but not the least; I thank my family for being a constant source of support in all my research endeavours.

Editor

HIV and Altered Immune Responses

Role of Dendritic Cell Subsets on HIV-Specific Immunity

Wilfried Posch, Cornelia Lass-Flörl and
Doris Wilflingseder

Additional information is available at the end of the chapter

1. Introduction

DC are key regulators of immunity in view of the fact that they are involved in immune responses against infectious diseases, allergy and cancer [1, 2]. Ralph Steinman was awarded the Nobel Prize for Medicine 2011 for DC discovery in 1973 [3]. Steinman and Cohn [3] described a novel cell type in mouse spleen, which they named ´dendritic cell´ due to their tree-like shape. The major function of DC is the induction of adaptive immunity in the LN.Yet, DC can also interact with innate immune cells, for instance natural killer (NK) and NKT cells [1, 4].

Upon entry of HIV into the host, the virus has to be transported from mucosal surfaces to lymphatic tissues, where it is transmitted to its primary targets, CD4+ T lymphocytes. This process is thought to be contrived by DC.

DC thereby play critical roles during HIV and SIV (simian immunodeficiency virus) infection.

The skin and mucosa are composed of two compartments, the epidermis and the dermis (skin) or stratified squamous epithelium and lamina propria (mucosa), each containing a major subset of DC - Langerhans cells (LC) reside in the suprabasal layers of the epidermis and epithelia [5], while dermal/interstitial DC are distributed throughout the connective tissue of the dermis [6, 7].

Both subsets represent immature DC that are very efficient in Ag uptake and processing. As immature DC (iDC), they reside in peripheral tissue, which they survey for invading pathogens. Upon encounter with antigen (Ag), DC mature (mDC) and migrate to the draining lymph nodes (LN). They pass through different maturation stages, which enable them to fulfill specific tasks such as the uptake, the processing and the presentation of Ag on major histocompatiblity complex (MHC) molecules to naïve T cells. In the T cell area of lymphatic tissue the mature DC stimulate Ag-specific CD4⁺ and CD8⁺ T cells to proliferate and develop effector function, such as cytokine production and cytotoxic activity. Effector T cells are recruited to inflamed peripheral tissue and participate in the elimination of pathogens and infected cells. This very particular life cycle illustrates why DC are called the 'sentinels of the immune system' [8].

In humans, different DC subsets have been identified in blood, spleen and skin, but little is known respecting resident and migratory DC in human LN. This book chapter will review the major DC subsets found in humans and their role in HIV-pathogenesis. If data are available, also the role of the viral opsonization pattern and its impact on DC interaction will be discussed.

2. DC subsets and their role in HIV infection

DC are divided into two main groups: conventional myeloid DC (cDC) and non-conventional plasmacytoid DC (pDC) (Figure 1). As recently described byDoulatov et al. (2010) [9], human multi-lymphoid progenitors can bring forth all lymphoid cell types, including monocytes, macrophages and DC. Nonetheless, most DC in steady-state emerge from a common myeloid progenitor [10]. DC areheterogenous subtypes with distinct functions, properties and localization [11]. DC progenitors migrate from the bone-marrow through the blood to lymphoid organs and peripheral tissues. There, they give rise to different cDC subsets (Figure 1). LC display an exception within the cDC group since they maintain in the epidermis independent on circulating precursors [12]. Within cDC, migratory and lymphoid-resident DC are distinguished: migratory DC travel from peripheral tissues to lymphoid organs, whereas lymphoid-resident DC populate lymphoid organs during their whole life-span and lack the migratory function. In humans cDC comprise Langerhans Cells (LC), dermal DC (CD103⁺ and CD103⁻), BDCA1⁺ (CD1c)- and BDCA3⁺ (CD141) DC, and the recently described CD56⁺ DC (Figure 1). They are localized in the skin, secondary lymphoid organs (spleen, tonsils) and blood. pDC develop in the bone-marrow and then they reside in lymphoid organs [13]. HLA-DR⁺CD123⁺pDC express BDCA2 and this cell subset is found in blood, secondary lymphoid organs as well as peripheral tissues, e.g. skin or lungs (Figure 1). The cDC subtypes and pDC express a different receptor repertoir and comprise distinct functions with respect to HIV spread, antiviral activity and transmission, which is reviewed below and shown in Figure 1 (Table adapted from Altfeld et al., [14]). Both cell types are resident in lymphoid tissues in the steady state, but during an inflammatory response, pDC and cDC are actively recruited to these tissues [15-17].

2.1. cDC

2.1.1. LC and HIV

LC survey the basal and suprabasal layers of the stratified squamous epithelium of the skin and oral and ano-genital mucosa for invading pathogens [18-21]. Due to their ideal

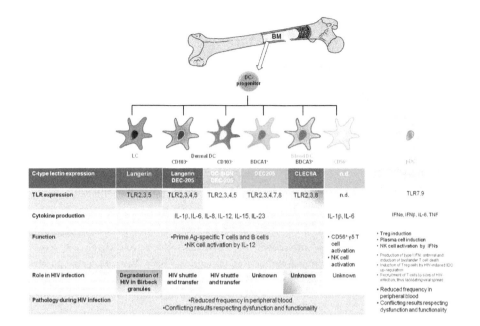

Figure 1. DC-subsets and functions during HIV-infection (Table adapted from *Altfeld et al., 2011*; CD56+ DC added). HIV co-localizes with Langerin in LC to high extend as shown by confocal microscopic analyses (co-localization: yellow). CD1a+ LC were isolated from human skin, incubated with HIV for 2 hrs, fixed and permeabilized with Cytofix/-perm (BD Biosciences). The cells were then stained using an anti-human Langerin-PE mAb (red, Dendritics) and the anti-HIV-Ab KC57-FITC ((green, Beckman Coulter). The nucleus was stained using DRAQ5™ (blue, Invitrogen) (*Posch et al., unpublished*).

localization in mucosal tissues and their long dendrites to efficiently capture Ag, they comprise the first line defense against mucosal infections. After Ag acquisition, LC start to mature, as represented by up-regulation of co-stimulatory molecules (CD80, CD86, CD40), MHC class I and II molecules, CD83 and CCR7 and down-regulation of Langerin and E-cadherin [22].

Due to CCR7 up-regulation, the mature LC migrate to the LN along a CCL19 and CCL21-leu (leucine isoform of CCL21) gradient to efficiently prime T cells there [23]. Beside initiating an effective adaptive immune response, LC were illustrated by DeWitte et al. [24, 25] to also have important functions with respect to innate immune responses. Beside a specific set of TLRs (TLR2, 3, 5) and high expression of CD1a, LC express Langerin and contain Birbeck granules that might be crucial to their innate function [21, 26-29] (Figure 1). The C-type lectin Langerin interacts with non-opsonized HIV-1 (Figure 2) and other pathogens such as fungi and bacteria, via fucose or mannose residues. Thereby degradation of HIV-1 in Birbeck granules is promoted and HIV-1 dissemination is limited [24].

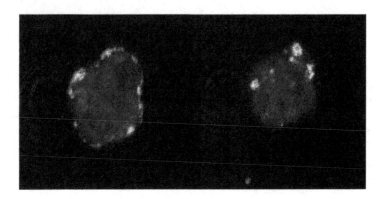

Figure 2. Co-localization of HIV and Langerin on CD1a⁺ Langerhans Cells isolated from human skin

Early investigations of HIV-LC interactions illustrated that LC are productively infected by HIV and that they efficiently transmit the virus to T cells [30-32]. These results suggested that HIV take advantage of the antigen-capturing properties of LC to reach the T cell zone in the lymphatic tissues and via this route, HIV can establish a productive infection of the host. However, *in vivo* only low percentages of LC are infected and despite abundant expression of the primary HIV-receptor CD4 and the chemokine co-receptor CCR5, high HIV-1 concentrations are required to infect LC *in vitro* [31, 32]. As shown by Wu and KewalRemani [33] the percentages to acquire HIV-1 after heterosexual contact with an HIV-positive individual are between 0.01 to 0.1%, which might be due to a restriction by LC.

Engagement of Langerin trimers on the surface of LC induces formation of Birbeck granules, which are part of the endosomal recycling system and uniquely found in LC (Figure 3, lower right panel) [34]. Upon capture of mycobacterial lipoproteins by Langerin, these were exposed to CD1a molecules in Birbeck granules [35], which suggests that Birbeck granule formation displays a non-classical antigen processing pathway [20]. Also HIV-1 attaches to Langerin on LC and is subsequently routed to Birbeck granules, which points to a role of the granules with respect to degradation of viruses.

Studies by Gejitenbeek's laboratory [24] showed that under homeostatic conditions, Langerin expressed on LC and acts as restriction factor for HIV infection. They demonstrated that, if HIV-gp120 attaches to Langerin, the viral particle is internalized and subsequently degraded in Birbeck granules. Thus, LC are protected from infection with incoming, non-opsonized HIV particles and HIV-1 is not disseminated throughout the host [24]. The rapid internalization of HIV-1 into LC by Langerin impedes interactions and subsequent fusion with CD4 and CCR5 and also prevents transmission to the main target cells of the virus, CD4⁺ T cells. Thereby, Langerin acts as a protective anti-HIV barrier during the first steps of HIV-1 infection, if the virus is non-opsonized and if sexually transmitted pathogens are lacking.

As demonstrated, if the host system is facing other sexually transmitted infections, the anti-HIV-1-barrier of LC is abrogated and HIV-1 transfer to susceptible CD4⁺ T cells is promoted [20, 36, 37]. Pathogens, such as Candida or Neisseria, directly interact with Langerin and compete with HIV-1-binding. Additional factors explaining the by-passing of the anti-HIV-1-barrier function of Langerin are that:

- by high viral loads the receptor becomes saturated,

- infections, e.g. Herpes simplex virus infection, down-regulate Langerin surface expression [20],

- the HIV-1 entry receptors CD4 and CCR5 are up-regulated during additional sexually transmitted infections [37],

- or the antiviral function of Langerin is reverted by inflammation-induced TNF-α (tumor-necrosis-factor α) production due to Candida albicans or Neisseria gonorrhoea [36].

These observations allow to conclude that during acute co-infection the anti-viral function of LC is significantly decreased.

Not only acute co-infection, but also opsonization of HIV with either complement fragments or specific Abs might result in reduction or abolishment of the anti-viral function mediated by Langerin (*Wilflingseder and Posch, unpublished data*). Upon entry of viruses into the body, immediate non-specific immune responses are triggered and within a short time the innate immune system is completely activated. During acute infection multiple humoral and cellular players, including cytokines, complement, acute-phase proteins, DC, macrophages, and natural killer (NK) cells, that co-operate to generate an efficient defense against infection, are activated. HIV-1 spontaneously triggers the complement system also in absence of specific Abs by interactions of gp41 with C1q [38-41]. Due to regulators of complement activation (RCAs) in the viral surface, HIV-1 is very efficiently protected against virolysis, which normally occurs due to MAC (membrane attack complex) formation and destruction of pathogens or infected cells. The incorporation of RCAs in the viral surface acts as protection mechanism and results in opsonization of HIV-1 with complement C3 fragments at the very initial steps following viral entry. After seroconversion, when HIV-1-specific Abs are established, the virus additionally is opsonized with specific IgGs. The different coating patterns of the virus change the receptor used on DC due to the density of complement fragments or Abs on the viral surface [42]. The C-type lectin-virus interaction becomes rather unimportant if the virus is opsonized and is substituted by complement or Fc receptor-virus interactions as already demonstrated using dermal DC [42]. After LC incubation using complement-opsonized HIV-1, we found that not only sexually transmitted diseases abrogate the antiviral barrier mediated via Langerin but also opsonization of HIV-1 (*Wilflingseder and Posch, unpublished data*).

In summary, during acute co-infection or by opsonization with complement fragments or Abs, the anti-viral function of LC is significantly reduced due to competition for Langerin or different receptor utilization. This facilitates HIV-1 infection of LC via CD4 and CCR5, intracellular uptake of the virus (Figure 3) and promotion of HIV-1 transfer to its targets, CD4+ T cells.

On the other hand LC were implicated in establishment of infection due to their location in the foreskin and due to compelling evidence that male circumcision efficiently reduces the risk to become infected with HIV-1 [43]. It was furthermore shown *in vivo* in highly HIV-1-exposed but (IgG) seronegative individuals, that gp41-specific IgA Abs efficiently blocked transfer of sexually transmitted HIV-1 [44-46]. A very recent study by Tudor et al. [46] illustrated that monomeric 2F5 IgA2 bound to gp41 MPER (membrane proximal external region) and free virus with greater efficiency than IgG1 and interferred with the initial HIV-1 transmission via Langerhans Cells. 2F5 IgA2 and IgG1 monomers blocked HIV-1 transcytosis in monostratified or multilayered epithelia as well as in rectal tissue [46, 47]. These Abs decreased infection of CD4+ T cells and transfer from LC to autologous CD4+ T cells [46]. The 2F5 IgA2 monomer inhibited virus transcytosis and CD4+ T cell infection more efficiently, while the 2F5 IgG1 monomer was superior in blocking the LC-CD4+ T cell transmission. A synergistic effect of both, 2F5 IgA2 and IgG1, was observed with respect to LC-CD4+ T cell transmission and decrease of CD4+ T cell infection [46].

2.1.2. Dermal DC and HIV

Along with LC, HIV-1 firstly attaches to dermal (interstitial) DC upon entry at mucosal surfaces (Figure 1). Dermal DC are underlying the epithelium, do not contain Birbeck granules and express heterogenous amounts of CD1a [48].

Interstitial DC are localized in the dermis and oral, vaginal and colonic lamina propria [6, 49-52]. They are characterized by the expression of CD11c, high expression of various C-type lectin receptors (Langerin on CD103+ DC, DC-SIGN on CD103- DC, DEC-205 on both subsets), TLR2, 3, 4 and 5 and they secrete various cytokines upon pathogenic stimulation (Figure 1). Since there are only 2 studies available on human CD103+ DC and SIV [53, 54], the following chapter refers to CD103-, DC-SIGN+ dermal DC.

In vitro experiments showed that DC efficiently capture HIV-1 or SIV, independent on the maturation status of the cells (Figure 3 and [55]) and subsequently transfer the virus to CD4+ T cells, which initiates a vigorous infection [41, 42, 56, 57]. These experiments imply that *in vivo* HIV exploits DC at mucosal sites as shuttles to CD4+ T cells in the LN, but the exact events with respect to virus spread from mucosal sites to LN have not been enlightened yet. Thereby, DC seem to play a significant role in the spread of infection as well as in the induction of antiviral immunity.

As shown in Figure 3, dermal DC (left panel) and LC (right panel), which emigrated from whole skin explants, take up variable amounts of HIV-1 particles. As demonstrated by Frank et al. [55], human and macaque DC interacted similarly with SIV and ample amounts of virus were captured by DC. Transmission electron microscopic analyses revealed that iDC, which are endocytically highly active, captured few viral particles near the periphery of the membrane, while mDC, which down-regulate the endocytic capacity, retained high amounts of virions in large vesicular compartments deeper within DC [55]. This points to a diverse entry and handling of virions within iDC and mDC.

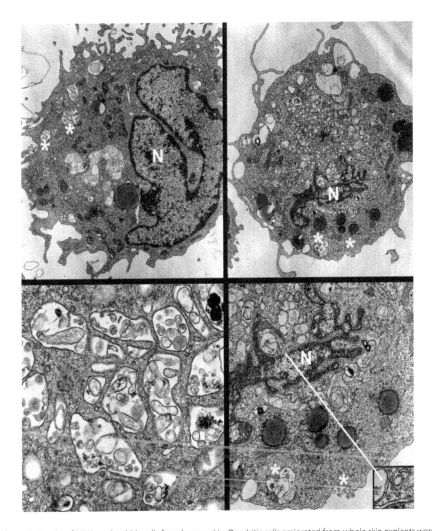

Figure 3. Uptake of HIV into dendritic cells from human skin. Dendritic cells emigrated from whole skin explants were incubated with HIV for 2h and then fixed and embedded for transmission electron microscopy. Variable amounts of viral particles are taken up by dermal dendritic cells (left panels) and epidermal Langerhans cells (right panels). Lower panels show higher magnifications of membrane-enclosed virus particles in a dermal dendritic cell (left panel; some viruses marked with red/black). In a Langerhans cell (lower right panel) viruses can be seen docking onto the surface membrane (right asterisk) and already taken up into vesicular structures (left asterisk). A Birbeck granule is depicted in the inset as the identifying structure for Langerhans cells. N, nucleus.(Photos courtesy of Hella Stössel and Nikolaus Romani).

Beside the different handling of HIV-1 or SIV within iDC and mDC, opsonization of the virus with either complement fragments and/or Abs significantly affects the binding mechanism, internalization and infection of DC as well as their T cell stimulatory capacity [41, 42, 58]. As shown by Pruenster et al. [42], the complement cloud around the virus significantly blocked the accessibility of gp120 and therefore interfered with C-type lectin interaction.

Similar amounts of HIV-1 bound to the surface of DC independent on the opsonization pattern of the virus (Pruenster et al., 2005). The attachment of the differentially opsonized HIV-1-preparations was found to be specific (Figure 4 [*Wilflingseder and Posch, unpublished data*]), since pre-incubation of the DC with blocking Abs against human DC-SIGN, CD11b (CR3-α chain) or CD32 (FcγRII) particularly blocked the interactions with the corresponding virus preparations:

• blocking α-DC-SIGN mAb inhibited interaction with non-opsonized HIV-1 (Figure 4, HIV),

• blocking α-CR3mAb (TMG6.5) significantly interferred with binding of complement-opsonized HIV (HIV-C) to DC (Fig.4, HIV-C) and

• blocking α-CD32mAb (AT10) inhibited binding of Ab-opsonized HIV-1 (Figure 4, HIV-Ig).

Additionally, we found variations respecting infection of DC with differentially opsonized HIV-1 preparations [41]. Productive infection of DC and LC with HIV-1 was described to be relatively inefficient compared to HIV-infection of CD4+ T cells and HIV- or SIV-infected DC are rarely detected *in vivo* (rev. in Piguet and Steinman[59]). Our study using non-, complement-, complement-Ig- or Ig-opsonized HIV-1 uncovered that complement-opsonization of HIV-1 significantly enhanced DC-infection compared to non-opsonized HIV [41] and furthermore acted as an endogenous adjuvans for DC-mediated induction of HIV-specific CTLs [58].

In contrast, HIV-1 coated with specific, non-neutralizing Abs significantly impaired infection of and integration in DC and also 'trans'-infection of CD4+ T cells after delayed addition of T cells [41].

Despite the low-level productive infection of DC, non-opsonized HIV-1 is very efficiently transmitted to T cells either via de novo ('cis'-transfer) or without ('trans'-)infection [60]. This is also true for Ab-opsonized HIV-1, if CD4+ T cells are added immediately to HIV-exposed DC [41]. Especially C-type lectins, such as DC-SIGN on dermal DC, were connected to transmitting HIV-1 to T cells in the LN [60, 61]. Similar to Langerin, DC-SIGN has high affinity for mannose and fucose structures, but despite sharing this feature these receptors exert completely different effects and functions regarding pathogen processing. Dermal CD103- DC express DC-SIGN, which captures low titres of HIV-1 by interaction with the envelope glycoprotein gp120 [62]. By complexing DC-SIGN via gp120, HIV-1 is protected from degradation within the DC in contrast to Langerin, which promotes degradation of the virus through Birbeck granules as described above [24, 62]. DC-SIGN-complexed HIV-1 remains stable and infectious over prolonged periods of time within non-lysosomal acidic organelles of DC [62, 63]. Thereby, DC-SIGN efficiently transfers HIV-1 to CD4⁺ T cells, enhances infection in DC-CD4⁺ T cell co-cultures and facilitates 'trans'-infection of the T cells [62].

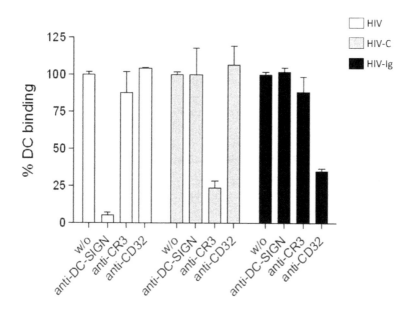

Figure 4. Binding of differentially opsonized HIV (non-opsonized HIV, HIV-C, HIV-Ig) in absence and presence of a blocking anti-human DC-SIGN, CR3 [CD11b] (TMG6.5) or CD32 (AT-10) antibodies. Binding of non-opsonized HIV was signficantly decreased in the presence of a blocking anti-DC-SIGN Ab, but not affected by pre-incubation of the cells with a blocking anti-CR3- or CD32-Ab (white bars). HIV-C-interaction with DC was inhibited using a blocking anti-CD11b (CR3)-Ab TMG6.5, but not by anti-DC-SIGN or CD32 (grey bars). Binding of IgG-opsonized HIV was inhibited by using a blocking anti-human CD32, but not DC-SIGN or CD11b-Ab (black bars).

Lastly, the antigen-presenting capacity of DC was also shown to be modulated by the opsonization pattern of the virus [58]. Earlier studies illustrated the role of complement opsonization respecting induction of effective CTL responses against viral infections, but the exact mechanism was not determined [64-66]. The exclusive role of DC in priming naïve CD8⁺ T cells in response to exogenous cell-associated as well as endogenously synthesized Ags has been shown [67, 68]. Endogenously synthesized antigens from DC infected with LCMV (choriomeningitis virus) mediated strong CTL responses, while macrophages and B cells infected with LCMV did not induce CTLs [68].

We recently found that opsonization of retroviral particles with complement fragments enhanced the ability of DC to induce CTL responses both *in vitro* and *in vivo* [58]. HIV-C-loaded DC mediated significantly higher CD8⁺ T cell expansion and signficantly better antiviral activity than DC exposed to non-opsonized HIV *in vitro*. This was further verified *in vivo* using the murine Friend virus model. These results indicated that 'complement acts as natural adjuvant for DC-induced expansion and differentiation of specific CTLs against retroviruses' [58].

Additionally, we demonstrated that in contrast to complement opsonization, antibody-coating of the viral surface attenuated the CTL-stimulatory capacity of HIV-exposed DC [69]. In some HIV-1-positive individuals, high levels of antibodies and low levels of complement fragments coat the HIV-1 surface and therefore we investigated the effects of the non-neutralizing Abs bound to the surface of HIV-1 on the CTL-stimulatory capacity of DC. We observed *ex vivo* and *in vitro* that DC loaded with IgG-opsonized HIV significantly impaired the HIV-1-specific CD8+ T cell response compared to the earlier described efficient CD8+ T cell activation induced by DC exposed to complement-opsonized HIV. These novel modulatory effects of the HIV-1-opsonization pattern on the CTL-activating capacity of DC might influence future vaccination strategies, since strong transient Ab responses subsequent to vaccination might weaken the CTL-induction by DC, which has to be considered [69].

Preferential expression of CCR5 on immature LC and DC restricts the transmission of X4-tropic isolates at the site of infection. Additionally, *ex vivo* analyses revealed that X4-tropic HIV replicate worse in DC and LC compared to R5-tropic viruses [31, 70, 71]. The relatively low susceptibility of DC to HIV-1-infection but efficient transfer of virus to CD4+ T cells was lately ascribed to an HIV-1 escape mechanism from innate recognition by DC [72, 73]. Manel et al. [72] showed that if DC by-pass resistance to HIV-1 infection [74, 75], they mature, exert a type I IFN response as well as adaptive immune responses. More recently, Laguette et al. [73] described the restriction factor SAMHD1 (SAM domain and HD domain-containing protein 1) to be responsible for inhibiting HIV-1 replication in DC and other cells of the myeloid lineage by degrading or preventing accumulation of HIV-1 DNA due to a putative nucleotidase activity. As shown by Lahouassa et al. [76], SAMHD1 depletes the pool of intracellular dNTPs and thus restricts HIV-1 infection in DC by blocking reverse transcription. These recent important findings respecting a formerly unknown cryptic innate sensor in DC, SAMHD1, and the induction of an efficient type I IFN and adaptive immune response due to DC infection might pave the way for novel therapeutical approaches to treat retroviral infections.

2.1.3. Blood DC and HIV

2.1.3.1. BDCA1+ DC, BDCA3+ DC, CD56+ DC and HIV

BDCA1+ myeloid DC can be directly isolated from human blood. This population was described to be reduced in the blood of HIV-infected individuals [76-78]. We found that BDCA1+ DC exerted a decreased transmission of HIV-1 to autologous CD4+ T cells, when the virus was opsonized with specific IgGs in contrast to non- or complement-opsonized HIV-1 and when the T cells were added delayed [41]. When CD4+ T cells were immediately added after washing the differentially loaded DC, the same infection efficiency was observed using HIV, HIV-C or HIV-Ig [41]. The two-phase transfer of HIV to DC as described above (*trans*-infection: by-passing of the virus from endolysosomal compartments, first 24 hrs; *cis*-infection: 'de novo' HIV-1-infection of DC before transfer to T cells) was also observable in BDCA1[+] DC, because non- and complement-opsonized HIV-1, which cause productive infection of DC, efficiently infected autologous CD4[+] T cells in short- and long-term co-cultures. BDCA1[+] DC exposed to IgG-opsonized HIV-1, which were not productively infected by the virus, were not able to promote long-term transfer of HIV-1 to susceptible T cells [41].

BDCA3[+] DC represent the human equivalent to mouse CD8α[+] DC and they are the major producers of IFN-λ in response to dsRNA poly I:C [80].As recently described by Dutertre et al. [81] using an 11-color flow cytometric strategy, circulating BDCA1[+] DC and BDCA3[+] DC counts were reduced in 15 viremic, untreated patients compared to 8 HIV-1-positive individuals under treatment and 13 healthy donors. By using this method, they illustrated that both blood DC subsets expressed characteristic lineage markers: BDCA1[+] DC expressed CD14, while particularly BDCA3[+] DC displayed CD56 on their surface. BDCA3[+] DC were shown to be more significantly down-modulated in viremic patients compared to controls [82] and it remains to be investigated by longitudinal studies, if combined antiretroviral therapy can restore the pool of circulating myeloid BDCA1[+] and BDCA3[+] DC.

Blood CD56[+] DC were recently described by Gruenbacher et al. [83] and comprise intermediate-sized lymphocytes with an HLA-DR[high], CD80[+] and CD86[+] expression profile. Upon cultivation they acquire DC-like morphology with increased levels of above mentioned surface markers. Upon stimulation, they are able to efficiently stimulate CD56[+]$\gamma\delta$ T cells, which results in secretion of IFNγ, TNF-α, and IL-1β [84]. The role of CD56[+] DC respecting HIV-1 infection and pathogenesis needs to be further investigated.

2.2. pDC and HIV

Plasmacytoid DC (pDC) (Figure 1) or type 1 IFN-producing dendritic cells are innate immune cells in blood, which are specialized in releasing massive amounts of IFNα and IFNβ upon viral challenge, including HIV-1 [83]. They constitute <0.2-0.5% of peripheral blood mononuclear cells (PBMC) [85] and in humans, pDC express the characteristic surface markers BDCA-2 (CD303, CLEC4C) and CD123 along with BDCA4 (CD304, NRP1), but they do not express CD11c, a marker of myeloid DC, or CD14 [86].

pDCs are key players of the innate immune response *in vivo* and they can prime adaptive immunity due to the afore mentioned production of high type I interferon levels, especially upon exposure to viral products [15, 83]. Upon stimulation with DNA or RNA viruses, they produce up to 1000-fold higher amounts of type I interferons than other cells [84, 87, 88]. The IFNα production in pDC by viruses represents a two-step process – uptake of viruses occurs due to recognition of envelope glycoproteins by C-type lectin receptors, e.g. mannose receptor or BDCA2, but induction of IFNα in fact starts in endosomal compartments by ligation of TLR9 or TLR7 [89-91]. Pathogenic single-stranded RNA or unmethylated DNA are mainly recognized by TLR7 and TLR9 expressed inside pDC [92]. Thus, the viruses have to be ingested by pDC into endosomes and NFkB- and MAPK signals through MyD88 must be stimulated [93]. Not only viruses, but also virus-infected cells can potently activate IFNα production from pDC [94]. Once activated, pDCs mature and produce large quantities of pro-inflammatory and antiviral cytokines [95-97]. pDC respond with high amounts of different IFNα subsets, IFNβ, IFNκ, IFNλ and IFNω on a wide range of enveloped viruses including HIV-1. They additionally produce pro-inflammatory cytokines TNFα, IFNγ and IL-6 as well as chemokines CXCL-10, CCL-5 and CCL-4 among others [98]. Thereby, pDC also act as a linker between innate and adaptive immunity.

Data by Zhou et al. [99] indicate that subsequent to HIV-1 challenge, signaling via TLR7 triggers autophagy and increased IFNα production from human pDC. The IFNα secretion mediated by an autophagy-dependent pathway may play an important role for T cell triggering during HIV-1 pathogenesis.

Beside acting as pro-inflammatory cells, pDC also provide negative regulatory signals and thus induce tolerance. pDC express IDO (indoleamine 2,3-dioxygenase) and PDL-1 (programmed death ligand; 1) which are associated with the negative modulation of T cell responses and regulatory T cell induction [100-102].

During acute HIV-1 infection, NK cells are recruited and activated by pDC to the sites of infection and to LN due to IFNα secretion [103, 104]. IFNα was demonstrated to increase the perforin levels in NK and CD8$^+$ T cells. At the sites of infection 'DC-editing' occurs by NK cells, since activated NK cells delete immature pDC to select for the more immunogenic mature pDC [105-108].Beside NK cell recruitment and activation, pDC-secreted IFNα promotes maturation and migration of other DC subsets. Due to their localization, it is unlikely that pDC are involved in HIV-1 capture, transport and transmission, but they are supposed to control HIV-1 in the acute phase of infection due to their immediate antiviral and NK priming activity.

Chronic exposure to HIV-1 leads to hyperactivation of pDC resulting in simultaneous type I IFN secretion and IDO expression. Thus, pDC concurrently exert cytotoxic and suppressive effects on T cells during chronic HIV-1 infection [109].

HIV-1 infection not only disrupts DC homeostasis within myeloid DC subsets, but also pDC homeostasis is defective during chronic HIV-1 infection. cDC and pDC are lost from blood, which correlates with high viral loads and low CD4$^+$ T cell counts [76, 110-113]. Deficiencies in pDC function were among the earliest observations of immune dysfunction in HIV-1 infection and some of the earliest studies of the 'natural IFN-α-producing cells' (i.e. pDC) illustrated that PBMC from AIDS patients were severely compromised in their ability to produce IFN-α *in vitro* after stimulation with the virus.

Cell death and/or a failure of bone marrow progenitors to differentiate into pDC might contribute to the loss of pDC from blood of chronically infected individuals. In non-pathogenic models of SIV infection, no depletion of blood pDC was observed [114, 115] and HIV-1-positive individuals, who are able to control infection (= long-term non-progressors) were also shown to have increased numbers of blood pDC [111].In contrast, it was described that during HIV-2 infection, which is highly attenuated compared to HIV-1 infection in humans, also the numbers of blood pDC is found reduced [116]. Thereby, the exact role of pDC depletion during HIV infection is not clear yet.

The depletion of cDC from the sites of infection was ascribed to a higher expression of CCR7 on the surface of cDC and a signfic antly increased CCL19 expression in LN of SIV-infected animals, thus suggesting that inflamed LN lure cDC away from the sites of infection early during progressive SIV infection [117]. A similar mechanism can be imagined for pDC, which are recruited to inflamed LN via CXCL9 and E-selectin [16, 118], but the pDC loss could also be due to direct infection, enhanced apoptosis or CD95 up-regulation [119-123].

Not only pDC numbers are decreased during on-going HIV-1 infection, but also the quality of the cells is suffering. They exert a reduced ability to migrate towards the CXCR4 ligand CXCL12 [124], they stimulate Treg cells to dampen HIV-1 immunity and they furthermore shift the Treg-Th17 balance [125, 126]. So far, interactions of differentially opsonized HIV-1 preparations with pDC has not been investigated.

3. Outlook: Impact of the HIV-1 opsonization pattern on DC function

As follows of investigations on HIV-1 in the last 30 years, antibody responses against the virus are not effective and cellular immune responses not powerful enough to suppress or even control HIV-1. DC, the prime inducers and regulators of immunity and tolerance, are crucial in designing modern vaccines [127-130]. Therefore, nowadays vaccine science shall combine established classical vaccine approaches with new attempts based on the expanded immunological knowledge.

Innate and adaptive immune responses are needed to generate efficient, long-lasting protection. Immediate innate responses involve activation of the complement system, ligation of pattern recognition receptors e.g. TLRs, C-type lectins, activation of NK cells, cDC and pDC, and type I, II, as well as III interferons. For viral clearance, the optimal balance between CD4$^+$ and CD8$^+$ T cells is required during the adaptive immune responses. Current HIV-1 vaccination strategies include the use of peptides or monocyte-derived DC exposed to chemically inactivated HIV-1 and aim in designing a vaccine efficiently inducing both, cellular and humoral immune responses [131-133]. So far, disappointing results have been achieved in clinical trials targeting either cellular [134, 135] or humoral immunity [136, 137]. The most prominent AIDS vaccine trial so far was the RV144 in Thailand [138], which evoked strong, but transient Env-specific CD4$^+$ T cell and Ab responses, but only weak HIV-specific CD8$^+$ T cell responses [131, 138].

HIV-1 induces immediate responses of the immune system upon entering mucosal surfaces. There, the complement system constitutes a first line of defense against the virus. Recently, we illustrated an important role for complement opsonization of retroviruses as an endogenous adjuvant for DC-mediated CTL-induction [58].

Efficient early CD8$^+$ T cell responses are crucial in controlling HIV-1 replication and their key role in HIV-1 control is additionally substantiated by association of certain HLA class I alleles and an improved disease progression [139-141]. In view of our very recent observations ([58], [69]), we propose that CD8$^+$ T cells are efficiently primed by DC during acute viral infection, particularly by enhanced infection of DC with HIV-C [41]. Thus, more efficient presentation of endogenously synthesized viral Ags via HLA-ABC [41], and ore efficient cross-presentation from incoming complement-opsonized HIV-1 are mediated. In contrast, Ab-opsonization of HIV-1 weakens the CTL-induction by modulation of DC function and might influence future vaccination strategies [69].

As shown by Lu et al. [142-144] *in vitro* and *in vivo*, DC exposed to chemically (aldrithiol-2, AT-2)-inactivated HIV or SIV induced a virus-specific CTL response. This response was strong enough to kill HIV-1-infected CD4$^+$ T cells [142], to control the viral load in SIV-infected monkeys [143] and HIV-infected individuals [144].. The decrease of the viral load in the HIV-1-infected patients was associated with a higher amount of HIV-1-gag-specific CD8$^+$ T cells and HIV-1-specific CD4$^+$ T cells.

LC were described to allow more cross-priming of CD8$^+$ T cells, while dermal DC are more specialized in primingnaive CD4$^+$ T cells [145]. The finding that complement-opsonization of HIV prior loading of DC significantly enhanced the CD8$^+$ T cell-stimulatory capacity of the cells in combination with using specific DC subtypes might efficiently improve future vaccination strategies and there is good reason to address DC of the skin, especially Langerhans cells, for purposes of vaccination.

A greater understanding of the innate and adaptive processes and the different functions of DC subsets to HIV-1 infection will lead to development of an effective vaccine.

Acknowledgements

The authors would like to thank Nikolaus Romani and Hella Stössl for providing the transmission electron microscopic picture.

The work of the authors is supported by the Austrian Science Fund [FWF, P22165 and P24598 to DW], the Tyrolean Science Fund [TWF, project: D-155140-016-011 to WP] and the OeNB [project: 14875 to WP].

Author details

Wilfried Posch, Cornelia Lass-Flörl and Doris Wilflingseder

Innsbruck Medical University, Division of Hygiene and Medical Microbiology, Innsbruck, Austria

References

[1] Steinman RM, Hemmi H. Dendritic cells: translating innate to adaptive immunity. Curr Top Microbiol Immunol 2006; 311:17-58.

[2] Steinman RM, Idoyaga J. Features of the dendritic cell lineage. Immunol Rev 2010; 234:5-17.

[3] Steinman RM, Cohn ZA. Identification of a novel cell type in peripheral lymphoid organs of mice. I. Morphology, quantitation, tissue distribution. J Exp Med 1973; 137:1142-62.

[4] Fernandez NC, Lozier A, Flament C, et al. Dendritic cells directly trigger NK cell functions: cross-talk relevant in innate anti-tumor immune responses in vivo. Nat Med 1999; 5:405-11.

[5] Romani N, Holzmann S, Tripp CH, Koch F, Stoitzner P. Langerhans cells - dendritic cells of the epidermis. APMIS 2003; 111:725-40.

[6] McLellan AD, Heiser A, Sorg RV, Fearnley DB, Hart DN. Dermal dendritic cells associated with T lymphocytes in normal human skin display an activated phenotype. J Invest Dermatol 1998; 111:841-9.

[7] Dupasquier M, Stoitzner P, van Oudenaren A, Romani N, Leenen PJ. Macrophages and dendritic cells constitute a major subpopulation of cells in the mouse dermis. J Invest Dermatol 2004; 123:876-9.

[8] Banchereau J, Steinman RM. Dendritic cells and the control of immunity. Nature 1998; 392:245-52.

[9] Doulatov S, Notta F, Eppert K, Nguyen LT, Ohashi PS, Dick JE. Revised map of the human progenitor hierarchy shows the origin of macrophages and dendritic cells in early lymphoid development. Nat Immunol 2010; 11:585-93.

[10] Schlenner SM, Madan V, Busch K, et al. Fate mapping reveals separate origins of T cells and myeloid lineages in the thymus. Immunity 2010; 32:426-36.

[11] Heath WR, Carbone FR. Dendritic cell subsets in primary and secondary T cell responses at body surfaces. Nat Immunol 2009; 10:1237-44.

[12] Merad M, Manz MG. Dendritic cell homeostasis. Blood 2009; 113:3418-27.

[13] Randolph GJ, Ochando J, Partida-Sanchez S. Migration of dendritic cell subsets and their precursors. Annu Rev Immunol 2008; 26:293-316.

[14] Altfeld M, Fadda L, Frleta D, Bhardwaj N. DCs and NK cells: critical effectors in the immune response to HIV-1. Nat Rev Immunol 2011; 11:176-86.

[15] Cella M, Jarrossay D, Facchetti F, et al. Plasmacytoid monocytes migrate to inflamed lymph nodes and produce large amounts of type I interferon. Nat Med 1999; 5:919-23.

[16] Yoneyama H, Matsuno K, Zhang Y, et al. Evidence for recruitment of plasmacytoid dendritic cell precursors to inflamed lymph nodes through high endothelial venules. Int Immunol 2004; 16:915-28.

[17] Yoneyama H, Matsuno K, Toda E, et al. Plasmacytoid DCs help lymph node DCs to induce anti-HSV CTLs. J Exp Med 2005; 202:425-35.

[18] Katz SI, Tamaki K, Sachs DH. Epidermal Langerhans cells are derived from cells originating in bone marrow. Nature 1979; 282:324-6.

[19] Romani N, Stingl G, Tschachler E, et al. The Thy-1-bearing cell of murine epidermis. A distinctive leukocyte perhaps related to natural killer cells. J Exp Med 1985; 161:1368-83.

[20] de Jong MA, Geijtenbeek TB. Langerhans cells in innate defense against pathogens. Trends Immunol 2010; 31:452-9.

[21] Romani N, Clausen BE, Stoitzner P. Langerhans cells and more: langerin-expressing dendritic cell subsets in the skin. Immunol Rev 2010; 234:120-41.

[22] Merad M, Ginhoux F, Collin M. Origin, homeostasis and function of Langerhans cells and other langerin-expressing dendritic cells. Nat Rev Immunol 2008; 8:935-47.

[23] Villablanca EJ, Mora JR. A two-step model for Langerhans cell migration to skin-draining LN. Eur J Immunol 2008; 38:2975-80.

[24] de Witte L, Nabatov A, Pion M, et al. Langerin is a natural barrier to HIV-1 transmission by Langerhans cells. Nat Med 2007; 13:367-71.

[25] de Witte L, Nabatov A, Geijtenbeek TB. Distinct roles for DC-SIGN+-dendritic cells and Langerhans cells in HIV-1 transmission. Trends Mol Med 2008; 14:12-9.

[26] Valladeau J, Ravel O, Dezutter-Dambuyant C, et al. Langerin, a novel C-type lectin specific to Langerhans cells, is an endocytic receptor that induces the formation of Birbeck granules. Immunity 2000; 12:71-81.

[27] Liu YJ. Dendritic cell subsets and lineages, and their functions in innate and adaptive immunity. Cell 2001; 106:259-62.

[28] Flacher V, Bouschbacher M, Verronese E, et al. Human Langerhans cells express a specific TLR profile and differentially respond to viruses and Gram-positive bacteria. J Immunol 2006; 177:7959-67.

[29] Fahrbach KM, Barry SM, Ayehunie S, Lamore S, Klausner M, Hope TJ. Activated CD34-derived Langerhans cells mediate transinfection with human immunodeficiency virus. J Virol 2007; 81:6858-68.

[30] Blauvelt A, Glushakova S, Margolis LB. HIV-infected human Langerhans cells transmit infection to human lymphoid tissue ex vivo. AIDS 2000; 14:647-51.

[31] Kawamura T, Azuma M, Kayagaki N, Shimada S, Yagita H, Okumura K. Fas/Fas ligand-mediated apoptosis of murine Langerhans cells. J Dermatol Sci 2000; 22:96-101.

[32] Kawamura T, Qualbani M, Thomas EK, Orenstein JM, Blauvelt A. Low levels of productive HIV infection in Langerhans cell-like dendritic cells differentiated in the

presence of TGF-beta1 and increased viral replication with CD40 ligand-induced maturation. Eur J Immunol 2001; 31:360-8.

[33] Wu L, KewalRamani VN. Dendritic-cell interactions with HIV: infection and viral dissemination. Nat Rev Immunol 2006; 6:859-68.

[34] Birbeck MS. Electron microscopy of melanocytes. Br Med Bull 1962; 18:220-2.

[35] Hunger RE, Sieling PA, Ochoa MT, et al. Langerhans cells utilize CD1a and langerin to efficiently present nonpeptide antigens to T cells. J Clin Invest 2004; 113:701-8.

[36] de Jong MA, de Witte L, Oudhoff MJ, Gringhuis SI, Gallay P, Geijtenbeek TB. TNF-alpha and TLR agonists increase susceptibility to HIV-1 transmission by human Langerhans cells ex vivo. J Clin Invest 2008; 118:3440-52.

[37] Ogawa Y, Kawamura T, Kimura T, Ito M, Blauvelt A, Shimada S. Gram-positive bacteria enhance HIV-1 susceptibility in Langerhans cells, but not in dendritic cells, via Toll-like receptor activation. Blood 2009; 113:5157-66.

[38] 38. Ebenbichler CF, Thielens NM, Vornhagen R, Marschang P, Arlaud GJ, Dierich MP. Human immunodeficiency virus type 1 activates the classical pathway of complement by direct C1 binding through specific sites in the transmembrane glycoprotein gp41. J Exp Med 1991; 174:1417-24.

[39] Spear GT, Jiang HX, Sullivan BL, Gewurz H, Landay AL, Lint TF. Direct binding of complement component C1q to human immunodeficiency virus (HIV) and human T lymphotrophic virus-I (HTLV-I) coinfected cells. AIDS Res Hum Retroviruses 1991; 7:579-85.

[40] Stoiber H, Clivio A, Dierich MP. Role of complement in HIV infection. Annu Rev Immunol 1997; 15:649-74.

[41] Wilflingseder D, Banki Z, Garcia E, et al. IgG opsonization of HIV impedes provirus formation in and infection of dendritic cells and subsequent long-term transfer to T cells. J Immunol 2007; 178:7840-8.

[42] Pruenster M, Wilflingseder D, Banki Z, et al. C-type lectin-independent interaction of complement opsonized HIV with monocyte-derived dendritic cells. Eur J Immunol 2005; 35:2691-8.

[43] Auvert B, Taljaard D, Lagarde E, Sobngwi-Tambekou J, Sitta R, Puren A. Randomized, controlled intervention trial of male circumcision for reduction of HIV infection risk: the ANRS 1265 Trial. PLoS Med 2005; 2:e298.

[44] Mazzoli S, Trabattoni D, Lo Caputo S, et al. HIV-specific mucosal and cellular immunity in HIV-seronegative partners of HIV-seropositive individuals. Nat Med 1997; 3:1250-7.

[45] Tudor D, Derrien M, Diomede L, et al. HIV-1 gp41-specific monoclonal mucosal IgAs derived from highly exposed but IgG-seronegative individuals block HIV-1 epithe-

lial transcytosis and neutralize CD4(+) cell infection: an IgA gene and functional analysis. Mucosal Immunol 2009; 2:412-26.

[46] Tudor D, Yu H, Maupetit J, et al. Isotype modulates epitope specificity, affinity, and antiviral activities of anti-HIV-1 human broadly neutralizing 2F5 antibody. Proc Natl Acad Sci U S A 2012; 109:12680-5.

[47] Shen R, Drelichman ER, Bimczok D, et al. GP41-specific antibody blocks cell-free HIV type 1 transcytosis through human rectal mucosa and model colonic epithelium. J Immunol 2010; 184:3648-55.

[48] Bell D, Young JW, Banchereau J. Dendritic cells. Adv Immunol 1999; 72:255-324.

[49] Pavli P, Woodhams CE, Doe WF, Hume DA. Isolation and characterization of antigen-presenting dendritic cells from the mouse intestinal lamina propria. Immunology 1990; 70:40-7.

[50] Pavli P, Hume DA, Van De Pol E, Doe WF. Dendritic cells, the major antigen-presenting cells of the human colonic lamina propria. Immunology 1993; 78:132-41.

[51] Lenz A, Heine M, Schuler G, Romani N. Human and murine dermis contain dendritic cells. Isolation by means of a novel method and phenotypical and functional characterization. J Clin Invest 1993; 92:2587-96.

[52] Nestle FO, Zheng XG, Thompson CB, Turka LA, Nickoloff BJ. Characterization of dermal dendritic cells obtained from normal human skin reveals phenotypic and functionally distinctive subsets. J Immunol 1993; 151:6535-45.

[53] Klatt NR, Estes JD, Sun X, et al. Loss of mucosal CD103+ DCs and IL-17+ and IL-22+ lymphocytes is associated with mucosal damage in SIV infection. Mucosal Immunol 2012.

[54] Presicce P, Shaw JM, Miller CJ, Shacklett BL, Chougnet CA. Myeloid dendritic cells isolated from tissues of SIV-infected Rhesus macaques promote the induction of regulatory T cells. AIDS 2012; 26:263-73.

[55] Frank I, Piatak M, Jr., Stoessel H, et al. Infectious and whole inactivated simian immunodeficiency viruses interact similarly with primate dendritic cells (DCs): differential intracellular fate of virions in mature and immature DCs. J Virol 2002; 76:2936-51.

[56] Pope M, Gezelter S, Gallo N, Hoffman L, Steinman RM. Low levels of HIV-1 infection in cutaneous dendritic cells promote extensive viral replication upon binding to memory CD4+ T cells. J Exp Med 1995; 182:2045-56.

[57] McDonald D, Wu L, Bohks SM, KewalRamani VN, Unutmaz D, Hope TJ. Recruitment of HIV and its receptors to dendritic cell-T cell junctions. Science 2003; 300:1295-7.

[58] Banki Z, Posch W, Ejaz A, et al. Complement as an endogenous adjuvant for dendritic cell-mediated induction of retrovirus-specific CTLs. PLoS Pathog 2010; 6:e1000891.

[59] Piguet V, Steinman RM. The interaction of HIV with dendritic cells: outcomes and pathways. Trends Immunol 2007; 28:503-10.

[60] Turville SG, Santos JJ, Frank I, et al. Immunodeficiency virus uptake, turnover, and 2-phase transfer in human dendritic cells. Blood 2004; 103:2170-9.

[61] Geijtenbeek TB, van Vliet SJ, Engering A, t Hart BA, van Kooyk Y. Self- and nonself-recognition by C-type lectins on dendritic cells. Annu Rev Immunol 2004; 22:33-54.

[62] Geijtenbeek TB, Kwon DS, Torensma R, et al. DC-SIGN, a dendritic cell-specific HIV-1-binding protein that enhances trans-infection of T cells. Cell 2000; 100:587-97.

[63] Engering A, Geijtenbeek TB, van Kooyk Y. Immune escape through C-type lectins on dendritic cells. Trends Immunol 2002; 23:480-5.

[64] Kopf M, Abel B, Gallimore A, Carroll M, Bachmann MF. Complement component C3 promotes T-cell priming and lung migration to control acute influenza virus infection. Nat Med 2002; 8:373-8.

[65] Suresh M, Molina H, Salvato MS, Mastellos D, Lambris JD, Sandor M. Complement component 3 is required for optimal expansion of CD8 T cells during a systemic viral infection. J Immunol 2003; 170:788-94.

[66] Mehlhop E, Diamond MS. Protective immune responses against West Nile virus are primed by distinct complement activation pathways. J Exp Med 2006; 203:1371-81.

[67] Jung S, Unutmaz D, Wong P, et al. In vivo depletion of CD11c+ dendritic cells abrogates priming of CD8+ T cells by exogenous cell-associated antigens. Immunity 2002; 17:211-20.

[68] Probst HC, van den Broek M. Priming of CTLs by lymphocytic choriomeningitis virus depends on dendritic cells. J Immunol 2005; 174:3920-4.

[69] Posch W, Cardinaud S, Hamimi C, Fletcher A, Mühlbacher A, Loacker K, Eichberger P, Dierich MP, Pancino G, Lass-Flörl C, Moris A, Saez-Cirion A, Wilflingseder D. Antibodies attenuate the capacity of dendritic cells to stimulate HIV-specific CTLs. J All Clin Imm 2012; accepted

[70] Granelli-Piperno A, Delgado E, Finkel V, Paxton W, Steinman RM. Immature dendritic cells selectively replicate macrophagetropic (M-tropic) human immunodeficiency virus type 1, while mature cells efficiently transmit both M- and T-tropic virus to T cells. J Virol 1998; 72:2733-7.

[71] Ganesh L, Leung K, Lore K, et al. Infection of specific dendritic cells by CCR5-tropic human immunodeficiency virus type 1 promotes cell-mediated transmission of virus resistant to broadly neutralizing antibodies. J Virol 2004; 78:11980-7.

[72] Manel N, Hogstad B, Wang Y, Levy DE, Unutmaz D, Littman DR. A cryptic sensor for HIV-1 activates antiviral innate immunity in dendritic cells. Nature 2010; 467:214-7.

[73] Laguette N, Sobhian B, Casartelli N, et al. SAMHD1 is the dendritic- and myeloid-cell-specific HIV-1 restriction factor counteracted by Vpx. Nature 2011; 474:654-7.

[74] Mangeot PE, Duperrier K, Negre D, et al. High levels of transduction of human dendritic cells with optimized SIV vectors. Mol Ther 2002; 5:283-90.

[75] Goujon C, Jarrosson-Wuilleme L, Bernaud J, Rigal D, Darlix JL, Cimarelli A. With a little help from a friend: increasing HIV transduction of monocyte-derived dendritic cells with virion-like particles of SIV(MAC). Gene Ther 2006; 13:991-4.

[76] Lahouassa H, Daddacha W, Hofmann H, et al. SAMHD1 restricts the replication of human immunodeficiency virus type 1 by depleting the intracellular pool of deoxynucleoside triphosphates. Nat Immunol 2012; 13:223-8.

[77] Grassi F, Hosmalin A, McIlroy D, Calvez V, Debre P, Autran B. Depletion in blood CD11c-positive dendritic cells from HIV-infected patients. AIDS 1999; 13:759-66.

[78] Donaghy H, Pozniak A, Gazzard B, et al. Loss of blood CD11c(+) myeloid and CD11c(-) plasmacytoid dendritic cells in patients with HIV-1 infection correlates with HIV-1 RNA virus load. Blood 2001; 98:2574-6.

[79] Pacanowski J, Kahi S, Baillet M, et al. Reduced blood CD123+ (lymphoid) and CD11c + (myeloid) dendritic cell numbers in primary HIV-1 infection. Blood 2001; 98:3016-21.

[80] Luci C, Anjuere F. IFN-lambdas and BDCA3+/CD8alpha+ dendritic cells: towards the design of novel vaccine adjuvants? Expert Rev Vaccines 2011; 10:159-61.

[81] Dutertre CA, Amraoui S, Derosa A, et al. Pivotal role of M-DC8+ monocytes from viremic HIV-infected patients in TNFalpha over-production in response to microbial products. Blood 2012.

[82] Chehimi J, Campbell DE, Azzoni L, et al. Persistent decreases in blood plasmacytoid dendritic cell number and function despite effective highly active antiretroviral therapy and increased blood myeloid dendritic cells in HIV-infected individuals. J Immunol 2002; 168:4796-801.

[83] Gruenbacher G, Gander H, Rahm A, Nussbaumer W, Romani N, Thurnher M. CD56+ human blood dendritic cells effectively promote TH1-type gammadelta T-cell responses. Blood 2009; 114:4422-31.

[84] Siegal FP, Kadowaki N, Shodell M, et al. The nature of the principal type 1 interferon-producing cells in human blood. Science 1999; 284:1835-7.

[85] Tversky JR, Le TV, Bieneman AP, Chichester KL, Hamilton RG, Schroeder JT. Human blood dendritic cells from allergic subjects have impaired capacity to produce interferon-alpha via Toll-like receptor 9. Clin Exp Allergy 2008; 38:781-8.

[86] O'Doherty U, Peng M, Gezelter S, et al. Human blood contains two subsets of dendritic cells, one immunologically mature and the other immature. Immunology 1994; 82:487-93.

[87]   Fanning SL, George TC, Feng D, et al. Receptor cross-linking on human plasmacy-toid dendritic cells leads to the regulation of IFN-alpha production. J Immunol 2006; 177:5829-39.

[88]   Fitzgerald-Bocarsly P, Dai J, Singh S. Plasmacytoid dendritic cells and type I IFN: 50 years of convergent history. Cytokine Growth Factor Rev 2008; 19:3-19.

[89]   Milone MC, Fitzgerald-Bocarsly P. The mannose receptor mediates induction of IFN-alpha in peripheral blood dendritic cells by enveloped RNA and DNA viruses. J Immunol 1998; 161:2391-9.

[90]   Dzionek A, Sohma Y, Nagafune J, et al. BDCA-2, a novel plasmacytoid dendritic cell-specific type II C-type lectin, mediates antigen capture and is a potent inhibitor of in-terferon alpha/beta induction. J Exp Med 2001; 194:1823-34.

[91]   Krug A, French AR, Barchet W, et al. TLR9-dependent recognition of MCMV by IPC and DC generates coordinated cytokine responses that activate antiviral NK cell function. Immunity 2004; 21:107-19.

[92]   Hemmi H, Kaisho T, Takeuchi O, et al. Small anti-viral compounds activate immune cells via the TLR7 MyD88-dependent signaling pathway. Nat Immunol 2002; 3:196-200.

[93]   Gill MA, Bajwa G, George TA, et al. Counterregulation between the FcepsilonRI pathway and antiviral responses in human plasmacytoid dendritic cells. J Immunol 2010; 184:5999-6006.

[94]   Beignon AS, McKenna K, Skoberne M, et al. Endocytosis of HIV-1 activates plasma-cytoid dendritic cells via Toll-like receptor-viral RNA interactions. J Clin Invest 2005; 115:3265-75.

[95]   Kadowaki N, Antonenko S, Lau JY, Liu YJ. Natural interferon alpha/beta-producing cells link innate and adaptive immunity. J Exp Med 2000; 192:219-26.

[96]   Ito T, Amakawa R, Kaisho T, et al. Interferon-alpha and interleukin-12 are induced differentially by Toll-like receptor 7 ligands in human blood dendritic cell subsets. J Exp Med 2002; 195:1507-12.

[97]   97. Colonna M. Alerting dendritic cells to pathogens: the importance of Toll-like re-ceptor signaling of stromal cells. Proc Natl Acad Sci U S A 2004; 101:16083-4.

[98]   Fitzgerald-Bocarsly P, Jacobs ES. Plasmacytoid dendritic cells in HIV infection: strik-ing a delicate balance. J Leukoc Biol 2010; 87:609-20.

[99]   Zhou D, Kang KH, Spector SA. Production of interferon alpha by human immunode-ficiency virus type 1 in human plasmacytoid dendritic cells is dependent on induc-tion of autophagy. J Infect Dis 2012; 205:1258-67.

[100] Boasso A, Shearer GM. Chronic innate immune activation as a cause of HIV-1 immu-nopathogenesis. Clin Immunol 2008; 126:235-42.

[101] Boasso A, Vaccari M, Hryniewicz A, et al. Regulatory T-cell markers, indoleamine 2,3-dioxygenase, and virus levels in spleen and gut during progressive simian immunodeficiency virus infection. J Virol 2007; 81:11593-603.

[102] Chen W, Liang X, Peterson AJ, Munn DH, Blazar BR. The indoleamine 2,3-dioxygenase pathway is essential for human plasmacytoid dendritic cell-induced adaptive T regulatory cell generation. J Immunol 2008; 181:5396-404.

[103] Gerosa F, Baldani-Guerra B, Nisii C, Marchesini V, Carra G, Trinchieri G. Reciprocal activating interaction between natural killer cells and dendritic cells. J Exp Med 2002; 195:327-33.

[104] Megjugorac NJ, Young HA, Amrute SB, Olshalsky SL, Fitzgerald-Bocarsly P. Virally stimulated plasmacytoid dendritic cells produce chemokines and induce migration of T and NK cells. J Leukoc Biol 2004; 75:504-14.

[105] Portales P, Reynes J, Rouzier-Panis R, Baillat V, Clot J, Corbeau P. Perforin expression in T cells and virological response to PEG-interferon alpha2b in HIV-1 infection. AIDS 2003; 17:505-11.

[106] Portales P, Reynes J, Pinet V, et al. Interferon-alpha restores HIV-induced alteration of natural killer cell perforin expression in vivo. AIDS 2003; 17:495-504.

[107] Ferlazzo G, Tsang ML, Moretta L, Melioli G, Steinman RM, Munz C. Human dendritic cells activate resting natural killer (NK) cells and are recognized via the NKp30 receptor by activated NK cells. J Exp Med 2002; 195:343-51.

[108] Ferlazzo G, Munz C. NK cell compartments and their activation by dendritic cells. J Immunol 2004; 172:1333-9.

[109] Herbeuval JP, Shearer GM. HIV-1 immunopathogenesis: how good interferon turns bad. Clin Immunol 2007; 123:121-8.

[110] 110. Barron MA, Blyveis N, Palmer BE, MaWhinney S, Wilson CC. Influence of plasma viremia on defects in number and immunophenotype of blood dendritic cell subsets in human immunodeficiency virus 1-infected individuals. J Infect Dis 2003; 187:26-37.

[111] Almeida M, Cordero M, Almeida J, Orfao A. Different subsets of peripheral blood dendritic cells show distinct phenotypic and functional abnormalities in HIV-1 infection. AIDS 2005; 19:261-71.

[112] Killian MS, Fujimura SH, Hecht FM, Levy JA. Similar changes in plasmacytoid dendritic cell and CD4 T-cell counts during primary HIV-1 infection and treatment. AIDS 2006; 20:1247-52.

[113] Nilsson J, Boasso A, Velilla PA, et al. HIV-1-driven regulatory T-cell accumulation in lymphoid tissues is associated with disease progression in HIV/AIDS. Blood 2006; 108:3808-17.

[114] Mandl JN, Barry AP, Vanderford TH, et al. Divergent TLR7 and TLR9 signaling and type I interferon production distinguish pathogenic and nonpathogenic AIDS virus infections. Nat Med 2008; 14:1077-87.

[115] Campillo-Gimenez L, Laforge M, Fay M, et al. Nonpathogenesis of simian immuno-deficiency virus infection is associated with reduced inflammation and recruitment of plasmacytoid dendritic cells to lymph nodes, not to lack of an interferon type I re-sponse, during the acute phase. J Virol 2010; 84:1838-46.

[116] Cavaleiro R, Baptista AP, Foxall RB, Victorino RM, Sousa AE. Dendritic cell differen-tiation and maturation in the presence of HIV type 2 envelope. AIDS Res Hum Retro-viruses 2009; 25:425-31.

[117] Barratt-Boyes SM, Wijewardana V. A divergent myeloid dendritic cell response at vi-rus set-point predicts disease outcome in SIV-infected rhesus macaques. J Med Pri-matol 2011; 40:206-13.

[118] Sallusto F, Schaerli P, Loetscher P, et al. Rapid and coordinated switch in chemokine receptor expression during dendritic cell maturation. Eur J Immunol 1998; 28:2760-9.

[119] Patterson BK, McCallister S, Schutz M, et al. Persistence of intracellular HIV-1 mRNA correlates with HIV-1-specific immune responses in infected subjects on stable HAART. AIDS 2001; 15:1635-41.

[120] Fong L, Mengozzi M, Abbey NW, Herndier BG, Engleman EG. Productive infection of plasmacytoid dendritic cells with human immunodeficiency virus type 1 is trig-gered by CD40 ligation. J Virol 2002; 76:11033-41.

[121] Lore K, Smed-Sorensen A, Vasudevan J, Mascola JR, Koup RA. Myeloid and plasma-cytoid dendritic cells transfer HIV-1 preferentially to antigen-specific CD4+ T cells. J Exp Med 2005; 201:2023-33.

[122] Meyers JH, Justement JS, Hallahan CW, et al. Impact of HIV on cell survival and anti-viral activity of plasmacytoid dendritic cells. PLoS One 2007; 2:e458.

[123] Brown KN, Wijewardana V, Liu X, Barratt-Boyes SM. Rapid influx and death of plas-macytoid dendritic cells in lymph nodes mediate depletion in acute simian immuno-deficiency virus infection. PLoS Pathog 2009; 5:e1000413.

[124] Dillon SM, Robertson KB, Pan SC, et al. Plasmacytoid and myeloid dendritic cells with a partial activation phenotype accumulate in lymphoid tissue during asympto-matic chronic HIV-1 infection. J Acquir Immune Defic Syndr 2008; 48:1-12.

[125] Manches O, Munn D, Fallahi A, et al. HIV-activated human plasmacytoid DCs in-duce Tregs through an indoleamine 2,3-dioxygenase-dependent mechanism. J Clin Invest 2008; 118:3431-9.

[126] Favre D, Lederer S, Kanwar B, et al. Critical loss of the balance between Th17 and T regulatory cell populations in pathogenic SIV infection. PLoS Pathog 2009; 5:e1000295.

[127]   Steinman RM, Banchereau J. Taking dendritic cells into medicine. Nature 2007; 449:419-26.

[128]   Steinman RM. Dendritic cells in vivo: a key target for a new vaccine science. Immunity 2008; 29:319-24.

[129]   Ueno H, Schmitt N, Klechevsky E, et al. Harnessing human dendritic cell subsets for medicine. Immunol Rev 2010; 234:199-212.

[130]   Andrieu JM, Lu W. A dendritic cell-based vaccine for treating HIV infection: background and preliminary results. J Intern Med 2007; 261:123-31.

[131]   McElrath MJ, Haynes BF. Induction of immunity to human immunodeficiency virus type-1 by vaccination. Immunity 2010; 33:542-54.

[132]   Picker LJ, Hansen SG, Lifson JD. New paradigms for HIV/AIDS vaccine development. Annu Rev Med 2012; 63:95-111.

[133]   Buchbinder SP, Mehrotra DV, Duerr A, et al. Efficacy assessment of a cell-mediated immunity HIV-1 vaccine (the Step Study): a double-blind, randomised, placebo-controlled, test-of-concept trial. Lancet 2008; 372:1881-93.

[134]   McElrath MJ, De Rosa SC, Moodie Z, et al. HIV-1 vaccine-induced immunity in the test-of-concept Step Study: a case-cohort analysis. Lancet 2008; 372:1894-905.

[135]   Flynn NM, Forthal DN, Harro CD, Judson FN, Mayer KH, Para MF. Placebo-controlled phase 3 trial of a recombinant glycoprotein 120 vaccine to prevent HIV-1 infection. J Infect Dis 2005; 191:654-65.

[136]   Pitisuttithum P, Gilbert P, Gurwith M, et al. Randomized, double-blind, placebo-controlled efficacy trial of a bivalent recombinant glycoprotein 120 HIV-1 vaccine among injection drug users in Bangkok, Thailand. J Infect Dis 2006; 194:1661-71.

[137]   Rerks-Ngarm S, Pitisuttithum P, Nitayaphan S, et al. Vaccination with ALVAC and AIDSVAX to prevent HIV-1 infection in Thailand. N Engl J Med 2009; 361:2209-20.

[138]   McElrath MJ. Immune responses to HIV vaccines and potential impact on control of acute HIV-1 infection. J Infect Dis 2010; 202 Suppl 2:S323-6.

[139]   Carrington M, O'Brien SJ. The influence of HLA genotype on AIDS. Annu Rev Med 2003; 54:535-51.

[140]   Goulder PJ, Watkins DI. Impact of MHC class I diversity on immune control of immunodeficiency virus replication. Nat Rev Immunol 2008; 8:619-30.

[141]   Streeck H, Jolin JS, Qi Y, et al. Human immunodeficiency virus type 1-specific CD8+ T-cell responses during primary infection are major determinants of the viral set point and loss of CD4+ T cells. J Virol 2009; 83:7641-8.

[142]   Lu W, Achour A, Arlie M, Cao L, Andrieu JM. Enhanced dendritic cell-driven proliferation and anti-HIV activity of CD8(+) T cells by a new phenothiazine derivative, aminoperazine. J Immunol 2001; 167:2929-35.

[143] Lu W, Wu X, Lu Y, Guo W, Andrieu JM. Therapeutic dendritic-cell vaccine for simian AIDS. Nat Med 2003; 9:27-32.

[144] Lu W, Arraes LC, Ferreira WT, Andrieu JM. Therapeutic dendritic-cell vaccine for chronic HIV-1 infection. Nat Med 2004; 10:1359-65.

[145] Ratzinger G, Baggers J, de Cos MA, et al. Mature human Langerhans cells derived from CD34+ hematopoietic progenitors stimulate greater cytolytic T lymphocyte activity in the absence of bioactive IL-12p70, by either single peptide presentation or cross-priming, than do dermal-interstitial or monocyte-derived dendritic cells. J Immunol 2004; 173:2780-91.

Chapter 2

Immune Responses and
Cell Signaling During Chronic HIV Infection

Abdulkarim Alhetheel, Mahmoud Aly and
Marko Kryworuchko

Additional information is available at the end of the chapter

1. Introduction

The immune response can be defined by the reaction of the immune system to a particular antigen to which it is exposed. In order to understand immune responses against an infectious agent such as human immunodeficiency virus (HIV) and their regulation during the course of chronic HIV infection, we will provide a brief overview of HIV and its proteins and attempt to shed light on this disease process. We will also review the immune system, its components and describe how these components interact at the molecular levels to fight an invading pathogen such as HIV.

2. Human immunodeficiency virus (HIV)

AIDS (Acquired Immuno-Deficiency Syndrome) in patients was discovered in 1981 and characterized by the appearance symptoms including persistent lymphadenopathy and opportunistic infections such as Kaposi sarcoma, *Pneumocystis carinii* pneumonia. In addition, it was found that all of these patients shared a common defect in cell-mediated immunity characterized by a significant decrease in CD4+T lymphocytes, later revealed to be a principal target of infection [1-3]. Three years later, the causative agent of AIDS was identified as HIV [4, 5]. HIV was classified under the *lentivirus* genus and the *Retroviridae* family. It is an enveloped virus with a size of about 100 nm in diameter. Its genome consists of two identical copies of positive-sense single stranded RNA (ssRNA) that are reverse transcribed into cDNA in infected cells [2, 5]. Each ssRNA is about 9,500 nucleotides in length, and encodes three structural genes called gag, pol, env, and a complex of several other nonstructural regulatory genes known as tat, rev, nef, vif, vpr, and vpu [2, 5]. The gag gene encodes the viral structural proteins including p24 (capsid), p17 (matrix), p7 (nucleocapsid). The pol gene, on the other hand, encodes viral enzymes including p32 (integrase), p66 and p51 (reverse transcriptase), and p10 (protease). The env gene encodes the coat glycoproteins gp120 (surface) and gp41 (transmembrane), which play a major role in viral attachment and fusion with host target cell membranes. The nonstructural genes including transactivator of transcription (Tat), regulator of virion protein expression (Rev), negative regulatory factor (Nef), viral infectivity factor (Vif), viral protein R (Vpr), and viral protein U (Vpu) proteins, respectively, are also essential for viral replication and pathogenesis [2, 5].

3. The immune system and its cellular components

The immune system is a very complex and dynamic network, which can be broadly divided into innate and adaptive components [4,6,7]. The cellular components of innate immunity include dendritic cells, natural killer (NK) cells, NK T cells, macrophages, and granulocytes, whereas, the adaptive immunity is mediated by B and T lymphocytes [4,6-8]. The components of both branches act in conjunction and are regulated by soluble mediator proteins known as cytokines and chemokines in order to fight, clear, and protect the host from a wide variety of pathogens [4,6-8].

3.1. The innate immune system

The innate immune system is the first line of defense against invading pathogens. Viral infections including HIV induce the interferon (IFN) response that is characterized by the production and secretion of pro-inflammatory cytokines including type-I IFN (IFN-α/β). These cytokines have antimicrobial and anti-proliferative properties and serve to propagate the adaptive immune responses [9]. In humans, cellular RNA molecules are short stem secondary structures. In contrast, RNA viruses produce long dsRNA molecules in the infected cells as a part of their life cycle. Thus, the long dsRNA can be recognized as a foreign molecule and triggers both cellular and humoral innate immune responses [10]. There are two well charac-terized ways in which a cell can recognize pathogens. Distinct extracellular pathogen compo-nents are recognized by different Toll- like receptors (TLR) expressed on the cell surface or in the endosome such as TLR2, TLR3, TLR4, TLR7, TLR8, and TLR9 [11]. Intracellular replicating pathogens however, are recognized by RNA helicases, which are encoded by the retinoic acid-inducible gene I (RIG-I) and/or melanoma differentiation-associated gene 5 (MDA5) [12]. Following viral recognition, the activation and translocation of the transcription factor nuclear factor κB (NFκB) and interferon-regulatory factor (IRF)-3 to the nucleus occurs and promotes the transcription of IFN type I [13]. Production of type-I IFN stimulates the surrounding cells to produce a wide range of antiviral proteins including protein kinase R (PKR), myxovirus resistance factor, 2'-5' oligoadenylate synthase/RNaseL and dsRNA adenosine deaminase 1, which subsequently leads to the activation of eukaryotic initiation factor (eIF)-2, and transla-tion inhibition of both host and viral mRNAs [14].

Monocytes, which are the precursors of macrophages, as a part of the innate immune system, play a major role in controlling and clearing pathogens. They exhibit antimicrobial, antifungal, and antiparasitic properties [4,6-8]. They possess phagocytic and endocytic activity. In addition, they act as antigen presenting cells by uptaking, processing, and presenting antigen in the context of major histocompatibility complex (MHC) class II to CD4+ T cells. Moreover, they secrete inflammatory cytokines such as IFN type-I (IFN-α/β), interleukin (IL)-1, IL-6, IL-12, and chemokines such as IL-8 [4,6-8]. This stimulates the adaptive immune system and leads to the activation and differentiation of B and T lymphocyte populations. These important monocyte/macrophage (M/M) functions are largely driven and regulated by the responsiveness of these cells to numerous cytokines such as IFN-γ, IL-10, and Tumor Necrosis Factor (TNF)-α, and signals delivered to them via the TLR family through recognition of different microbial products such as bacterial lipopolysaccharide (LPS) and viral proteins and nucleic acids including those of HIV [4,6-8].

3.2. The adaptive immune system

B and T lymphocytes form the arm of the adaptive and antigen-specific immune response. B lymphocytes are antigen presenting cells, upon antigenic and cytokine stimulation they differentiate into plasma cells which produce antigen-specific antibodies. While T lymphocytes are divided into two distinct populations: helper and cytotoxic cells which are differ in their function T helper lymphocytes express the CD4 surface receptor, recognize antigens presented as peptide epitopes bound to MHC class II molecules expressed on the surface of antigen presenting cells, and function mainly as cytokine producing cells to 'help' the development of the immune response. Activated CD4+ T cells differentiate into T helper (Th)-1 and Th-2 effectors, and memory cell sub-populations. The Th-1 and Th-2 subsets of CD4+ T cells were originally defined by their polarized cytokine production patterns [15,16]. Th-1 cells produce IFN-γ, IL-2, IL-12 and lymphotoxin-α, which enhance antigen presentation, phagocytosis, and cell-mediated cytotoxicity. On the other hand, Th-2 cells secrete IL-4, IL-5, IL-9, IL-10, and IL-13, promoting more of an antibody response [16-18]. Cytotoxic T lymphocytes however, express the CD8 surface receptor, and recognize antigenic peptide epitopes presented on cell surface MHC class I molecules. Antigen-activated CD8+ T cells also proliferate and differentiate into effectors and memory cell populations, largely in response to cytokines that share the common γc receptor, such as IL-2, IL-15, and IL-7. Cytotoxic T cells secrete IFN-γ, which inhibits virus replication, as well as perforin, and granzymes in order to kill virus-infected cells.

3.3. HIV and the cellular immune response

HIV is commonly transmitted by sexual contact, and thus it initially interacts with and activates the innate immune system and antigen presenting cells including macrophages and dendritic cells at the mucosal surfaces [5,19,20]. Importantly, these cells then migrate to the lymphoid tissues and thereby also deliver the virus to other susceptible cells located at these sites. In the lymphoid tissues, HIV interacts and infects other cells such as CD4+ T cells and is able to disseminate to other areas such as the brain and gut [5,21]. Subsequently, inflammatory cells and cytokines accumulate during chronic infection and immune activation causing severe reactions and tissue pathology. This includes destruction of regulatory immune cells, mainly CD4+ T cells, and overall impairment of immune functions, which are the hallmarks of chronic HIV infection [5,22-24]. Studies have shown that M/M and T lymphocyte functions are impaired over the course of HIV infection, thus contributing to the overall immune dysfunction and appearance of the opportunistic infections observed in HIV-infected patients. Several *ex vivo* and *in vitro* studies have reported that many M/M defects arise during chronic HIV infection including poor phagocytic activity [25-27], altered cytokine and chemokine secretion [24,28-31], impaired antigen uptake and MHC class II molecule expression [32,33]. Other studies have shown defects in T lymphocyte effector functions including impairment of CD4 T lymphocytes to produce IL-2 and to proliferate in response to recall antigens (influenza, tetanus toxoid), alloantigens (mixed lymphocytes reaction), or exogenous mitogens (phyto-hemagglutinin) [34,35]. Also, CD8 T lymphocytes exhibit an altered differentiation and proliferative phenotype and impaired capacity to kill virus-infected cells and clear the virus [36]. However, the molecular mechanism by which HIV impairs these cellular functions remains unclear. One possible mechanism by which chronic HIV infection may adversely affect immune cell function is through the modulation of cell signaling molecules, as observed in several cell types including M/M, CD4+ and CD8+ T cells, and neuronal cells [37-42]. This may occur by the direct action of HIV and its different immunomodulatory proteins such as Gp120, Nef, Tat, and Vpr, or indirectly via its effects on the cytokine secretion profile induced during the course of the disease as discussed in more detail below [43-46].

4. Cytokines

As mentioned above, cytokines are small secreted proteins with molecular weights of about 10-40 kDa [18,47,48]. These proteins function as mediators to regulate both the innate and adaptive immune responses [4,6,7]. They transmit the biochemical message from the extracellular environment to the nucleus of the targeted cell via cytokine-cytokine receptor interaction and subsequent triggering of complex intracellular signal transduction [49,50]. They can affect cell function in a paracrine as well as an autocrine manner. There are many cytokines produced by the immune system. Certain cytokines are associated with the initial response to an infection or inflammation and are referred to as inflammatory cytokines. Other cytokines are induced according to the nature of the infectious agent and the type of immune responses produced against them. For instance, infection with *Influenza virus*, *Vaccinia virus*, or *Listeria monocytogenes* is known to induce a Th-1 immune response [51]. This type of immune response is associated with the production of cytokines such as IL-2, IFN-γ, and IL-12, which regulate cell-mediated immunity including delayed hypersensitivity reactions, activation of macrophages and leukocyte cytolytic processes, and result in the protection and elimination of intracellular pathogens [16,50,52]. On the other hand, infection with *Nippostrongylus barsiliensis* or *Leishmania major* is known to induce a Th-2 response [51]. This immune response is characterized by secretion of cytokines such as IL-4, IL-5, IL-9, IL-10, and IL-13 that predominantly regulate antibody-mediated immunity and generally lead to the protection and clearance of extracellular antigens/pathogens [16,50,52]. During chronic HIV infection, both types of immune response and their associated cytokines are dysregulated, which may result in altered M/M and lymphocyte functions and increased susceptibility to programmed cell death (PCD) [53-56].

The following section will focus on cytokines that play an important role in regulating M/M as well as T lymphocytes effector functions and cell survival. These cytokines include IFN-γ, granulocyte-macrophage colony-stimulating factor (GM-CSF), IL-10, IL-4, IL-2, IL-7, and IL-15 (summarized in Table 1).

Cytokine	Producer cells	Effects on M/M, T cells	STAT signaling in viremic patient
IFN-γ	Th1 lymphocytes, activated NK cells, and CD8 T cells	Upregulates the activation of MHC class I and II, and activates pathogen killing.	Increased STAT1 activation
IFN-α	Leukocytes, and virus-infected cells	Upregulates the activation of MHC class I.	Decreased STAT1 activation
GM-CSF	T cells, Macrophages	Stimulates growth and differentiation of myelomonocytic lineage cells. Enhances phagocytosis.	Not significantly affected
IL-10	T cells, Macrophages	Potent suppressor of monocytes/macrophage function (e.g. inhibits MHC class II activation, antigen presentation, and phagocytosis).	Not significantly affected
IL-4	Th2 lymphocytes	Induces activation of MHC class II, induces endocytosis, and mannose receptor activation.	Not significantly affected
IL-2	Activated T lymphocytes and dendritic cells	Promotes T cell proliferation and T reg development	Decreased STAT5 activation
IL-7	Bone marrow and stromal cells in lymphoid organs	Maintains thymocytes survival.	Decreased STAT5 activation
IL-15	M/M, dendritic cells, mast cells, epithelial cells, and fibroblast	Induces survival and proliferation of CD8 T cells, NK cells and NK T cells.	Not significantly affected

Table 1. Cytokines and their effects on monocyte/macrophage and T lymphocyte functions

4.1. Cytokines that affect monocytes

Cytokines such as IFN-γ and GM-CSF affect mainly M/M, while, IL-10 and IL-4 act on both M/M and lymphocytes. IFN-γ is an 18-kDa potent pleiotropic cytokine produced by NK cells, NK T cells, Th-1, and CD8+ T cells. It has a critical role in the regulation of both innate and adaptive immunity [57,58]. It inhibits Th-2 and promotes Th-1 cell polarization and differentiation. Also, it inhibits viral replication and regulates cell death [57,58]. Moreover, it activates monocytes and macrophages, increases MHC class II expression, promotes antigen processing and presentation, and enhances their phagocytic, antimicrobial, and tumoricidal activities [59-64]. For instance, it has been shown that treatment of M/M with IFN-γ enhanced phagocytic activity against many pathogens including *Aspergillus fumigatus*, *Cryptococcus neoformans*, *Listeria monocytogenes*, *Mycobacterium avium*, *Toxoplama cruzi and gondii* [26,61,65]. Other studies have revealed that the lack of IFN-γ responses, such as in IFN- γ, IFN-γ receptor (IFN-γR), or STAT1-deficient mice, or in patients with mutations in the IFN-γ-R gene, lead to impaired immunity and increased susceptibility to infection [66-70]. GM-CSF is a 22-kDa protein secreted by macrophages and T cells. It facilitates growth and differentiation of monocyte and granulocyte lineages. It also enhances M/M effector functions including phagocytic, antimicrobial and antiparasitic activities [71,72].

IL-10 is a potent immunosuppressive and anti-inflammatory cytokine produced by macrophages and T cells. It downregulates MHC class II molecule expression and antigen presentation to CD4+ T cells [73,74]. It also inhibits the expression of co-stimulatory molecules, B7.1/B7.2, on monocytes and macrophages as well as the production of various cytokines such as TNF-α, IL-1, IL-2, IFN-γ, IL-3, and GM-CSF [73,75,76]. In addition, it suppresses macrophage nitric oxide production, and anti-fungal activity [77]. Moreover, it stimulates proliferation and differentiation of B cells, and polarizes T cells towards a Th-2 type response [17,78].

IL-4 is a 20-kDa cytokine secreted by Th-2 lymphocytes that promotes a Th-2 immune response. It has dual immunoregulatory functions [18]. It activates B cell differentiation and antibody production. Also, it enhances macrophage cytotoxicity and their expression of MHC class II and mannose receptor [79-84]. On the other hand, it inhibits cytokine secretion such as TNF-α, IL-1, IL-6, IL-18, GM-CSF and granulocyte colony-stimulating factor (G-CSF) [85-94]. It also suppresses cytokine-induced macrophage activation, oxidative burst, and intracellular killing [62,95]. Moreover, it downregulates monocyte adhesion and CD14 expression [96,97], monocyte-mediated cytotoxicity, nitric oxide production, and anti-fungal activity [77,98].

4.2. Cytokines that affect lymphocytes

Cytokines that share the γ-chain receptor, such as IL-2, IL-7, and IL-15, play a critical role in lymphocyte growth and differentiation [36,99]. IL-2 is a protein produced mainly by activated CD4 but also CD8 T lymphocytes and dendritic cells. It is a T cell growth factor and plays a critical role in regulating the immune response. It plays a major role in activating the immune system in the presence of antigenic stimulation, but also in downregulating this response following pathogen clearance. IL-2 stimulates T cell proliferation and is essential for developing regulatory T cells. In addition, IL-2 has been shown to upregulate expression of Tumor Necrosis Family death receptor ligand, FasL, in activated T cells thereby enhancing their susceptibility to activation-induced cell death [100,101].

IL-7 is a pleiotropic cytokine secreted by bone marrow and stromal cells of lymphoid organs. It stimulates the growth and maintains the survival of thymocytes (B and T lymphocyte progenitor cells) by increasing the expression of the anti-apoptotic molecule Bcl-2 and downregulating the expression of the pro-apoptotic molecule Bax [102-105]. Thus, it is an essential element for T cell survival, proliferation, and optimal effector function.

IL-15 is a cytokine that is produced by different cell types including M/M, dendritic cells, mast cells, epithelial cells, and fibroblasts. It plays an important role in growth and homeostasis. It provokes adaptive and innate immune responses. For example, it shares several biological effects with IL-2 such as mediating survival and proliferation of naïve and memory CD8 T cells. It also stimulates NK T cell expansion and regulates the development of NK cells and its cytotoxicity [36,99,106].

It has been reported that during the course of chronic HIV infection, many inflammatory and anti-inflammatory cytokines such as TNF-α, IFN-β, IFN-γ, IL-18, IL-2, IL-10, and IL-4 are increased in patients serum [77,107-115], and thus may play a role in the alteration of M/M and T lymphocyte functions and signaling pathways (Table 1) [38-42]. Several studies have also proposed and used cytokines such as IFN-γ, GM-CSF, IL-4, IL-2, IL-7 and IL-15 as therapeutics in clinical trials for diseases including HIV and myeloma in an attempt to compensate for impairments in the cytokine network [36,99,116-118].

4.3. Cytokine signaling pathways

Cytokine signaling pathways can be defined as biochemical signaling cascades that are triggered within minutes to relay the information required to mediate various cytokine-dependent cellular functions [119-123]. Most cytokines share general mechanisms of signal transduction in which cytokine-cytokine receptor binding causes the assembly of the specific receptor subunits. Subsequently, a number of tyrosine kinases from the Src and Syk families are activated leading to signal transduction through mainly three major signaling pathways: (i) Janus Kinase (JAK)/Signal Transducer and Activator of Transcription (STAT), (ii) Phosphoinositide 3-kinase (PI3K), and (iii) Mitogen-activated protein kinase (MAPK) [124-126]. These signaling pathways form a very complex and evolutionarily conserved network.

A general overview of these cascades is illustrated in Figure 1. Briefly, when the ligand-receptor interaction occurs, subsequent events are activated based on the nature of these ligands and receptors. For example, a receptor with intrinsic kinase activity (e.g. epidermal growth factor receptor) is usually autophosphorylated directly leading to the creation of a docking site for an adapter protein complex called Grb2/SOS (son of sevenless) [36]. As a result, SOS is recruited to the plasma membrane where it encounters and activates a small G protein named Ras [36,127,128]. Activated Ras induces the activation of several downstream signaling molecules, including a serine/threonine kinase called Raf, which in turn activates the MAPK and PI3K signaling pathways [36,127,129]. PI3K signaling molecules can also be activated directly via the p110α catalytic subunit of the PI3K [127]. A receptor with no intrinsic kinase activity (e.g. cytokine receptors) generally requires activation of receptor-associated kinases such as JAKs for its phosphorylation. Subsequently, activated JAKs can activate the STAT signaling pathway directly and also interact with and activate Grb2/SOS, which in turn activates PI3K and MAPK signaling [36,122,130,131].

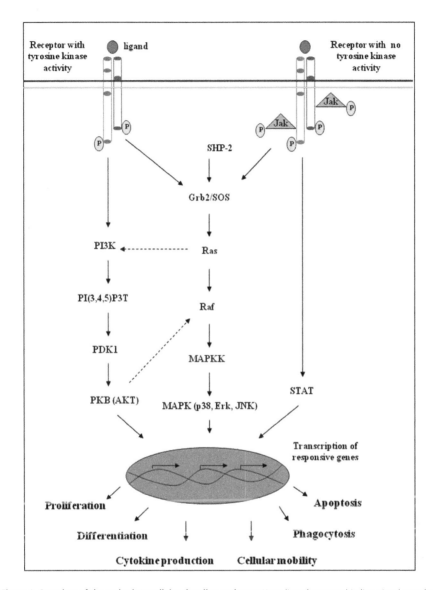

Figure 1. Overview of the major intracellular signaling pathways Upon ligand-receptor binding, signal transduction triggers takes place based on the type and nature of the receptor. If the receptor has intrinsic tyrosine kinase activity, autophosphorylation of the tyrosine residues of the receptor will occur and thus creates docking sites for a variety of different signaling molecules that have SH2 and PTB domains. Grb2/SOS complexes bind to docking sites and lead to recruitment of SOS (son of sevenless) to the plasma membrane where they interact with Ras. Subsequently, activated Ras molecules activate several downstream molecules including Raf, MAPKK, and MAPK. The PI3K signaling pathway can be activated directly via the p110α catalytic subunit of the PI3K. Phosphorylated receptors also

activate phospholipase Cγ (PLCγ), which activate Protein Kinase C (PKC) and calcium-dependent signaling pathways. If the receptor has no intrinsic kinase activity, activation of the Janus Kinase (Jak) or other receptor-associated kinase occurs. Subsequently, activated Jaks phosphorylate the receptor and thus create docking sites for various signaling molecules including members of the Signal Transducers and Activators of Transcription (STAT) family. Signal transduction culminates in the transcriptional activation of STAT responsive genes that influence cellular proliferation, differentiation, cytokine production, mobility, phagocytosis, and survival [modified from [187]].

Evidence has also demonstrated the presence of a complex crosstalk between these pathways. For instance, it has been shown that Jak2 is responsible for the activation of STAT, Erk MAPK, and Akt signaling pathways in response to growth hormone in hepatoma and preadipocyte cells [132]. Another report has demonstrated a role for Akt in serine phosphorylation of the STAT1 transcription factor and upregulation of gene expression in response to IFN-γ [133].

HIV-induced perturbation of the JAK/STAT, PI3K, and MAPK signaling pathways in immune cells including M/M and T lymphocytes has been documented (summarized in Table 1, 4) [41,134-146]. These effects appear to be to the advantage of the virus. On one hand, it may help the virus to replicate and establish infection. On the other hand, it may also help the virus to escape the immune system. In the following subsections, we will provide a brief overview of cytokine signaling and where HIV infection appears to target these cascades.

4.3.1. JAK/STAT signaling pathway

The JAK/STAT pathway is one of the major signaling pathways involved in cytokine responses. Studies have shown that many ligands such as epidermal growth factor (EGF), receptor tyrosine kinases (RTK), G protein-coupled receptors (GPCR) and several cytokine families including interferons and interleukins are the main triggers of the JAK/STAT signaling cascade [147-149]. An overview of the JAK/STAT signal transduction pathway is illustrated in Figure 1. Initially, cytokine-receptor interaction triggers tyrosine transphosphorylation of receptor-associated JAKs. This is followed by phosphorylation of receptor cytoplasmic domains by JAKs and recruitment of latent STAT proteins via their Src homology 2 (SH2) domains to the activated (tyrosine phosphorylated) receptor. This is followed by STAT tyrosine phosphorylation. Activated STATs form dimers via their SH2 domains and are translocated into the nucleus where they bind STAT responsive elements [119,120,123], and thus promote transcription of STAT responsive genes such as cytokine-inducible SH2-containing protein (CIS), members of the IRF family, and numerous other genes [150-153].

In mammalian cells, four JAKs (Jak1, Jak2, Jak3 and Tyk2) and seven STAT proteins (STAT1, 2, 3, 4, 5a, 5b, and 6) with their different isoforms have been identified. [147,154]. Through IL-6-induced signaling, Jak1 is the principal kinase in the downstream signaling cascade. It has been shown in many cell lines that down regulation of Jak1 would lead to impaired signal transduction. Activated JAKs lead to phosphorylation of STAT proteins. However, JAK kinases do not appear to show specificity for a particular STAT protein [147,154]. STAT proteins play an important role in regulating and maintaining both innate and adaptive immune responses (summarized in Table 2) [119-121,123]. For instance, studies have suggested that impairment of JAK/STAT signaling may increase susceptibility to many infections including HIV [65,67,70,155].

STAT gene	Activating cytokines	Examples of STAT responsive genes	Phenotype of knockout mice
STAT1	IFNs,IL-6,IL-10	IRF-1, ISG54, MIG, GBP, CIITA	Impaired IFN and innate immune responses, increase susceptibility to tumors, opportunistic and viral infections
STAT2	IFNs	IRF-1, ISG54	Impaired Type-1 IFN responses
STAT3	IL-2,IL-6,IL-10	JunB, SAA3, JAB, C-reactive protein, Bcl-xL	Embryonic lethal
STAT4	IL-12	IFN-γ, IRF-1, MHC class II, CD23, Fc-γRI	Defect in IL-4 and IL-12 responses, and impaired Th1 differentiation.
STAT5 a, b	Numerous (e.g. IL-2,IL-7,IL-15, GM-CSF)	CIS, IL-2R-α, β-casein, osm, pim1, p21	Impaired proliferation, growth and survival, defect in IL-2 responses, impaired growth.
STAT6	IL-4,IL-13	IL-4R-α, C-γ-1, C-γ-4	Defect in IL-4 responses, and impaired Th1 differentiation.

Table 2. STATs proteins and their role in the immune system

A number of reports have suggested that defects in cytokine responsiveness arise in different cell types during chronic HIV infection and these defects could be due to the direct effects of HIV and/or its proteins, or due to indirect effects associated with alterations of the host cytokine profile [38-42,139,141-143,156]. In M/M, it has been revealed that GM-CSF-induced STAT5 activation in monocyte-derived macrophages (MDM) is inhibited by *in vitro* HIV-1 infection [156]. Other *in vitro* reports have suggested that HIV and its Gp120 and Nef proteins are capable of activating STAT1 and STAT3 in monocytic cell lines and MDM [141-143]. Recently, the HIV matrix protein p17 has been shown to induce STAT1 and pro-inflammatory cytokines in macrophages [139]. Moreover, in *ex vivo* studies, we found that among the responses to cytokines tested (IFN-γ, IFN-α, IL-10, IL-4, and GM-CSF) in terms of STAT induction in monocytes, only IFN-γ showed a significant upregulation of STAT1 activation in HIV+ patients that were off antiretroviral therapy (ART) compared to HIV- controls and patients on ART [39]. Furthermore, this potentiation of IFN-γ-induced STAT1 activation was associated with increased total STAT1 expression levels and monocyte cell death [39]. Another *ex vivo* study has shown a defect in IFN-α induced STAT1 activation in monocytes obtained from a similar set of HIV patients, and this defect was due to the decreased IFN-α receptor expression levels on these cells [42].

In lymphocytes, we and others have shown that both IL-7Rα expression and IL-7-induced STAT5 activation was impaired in CD8 T cells from HIV+ patients [36,40,41]. STAT activation in response to IL-4 and IL-10 did not appear to be similarly impaired [40]. We also found that IL-2-induced STAT5 activation was inhibited in CD8+ T cells from a subset of HIV-infected patients naive to therapy, but was restored, at least in part, after ART [38]. Somewhat similar results have been observed in other *in vitro* studies in which activation of STAT5 in response to IL-2 was inhibited by HIV-1 infection through prior Gp120-CD4 interactions in CD4+ T cells [37,144].

4.3.2. PI3K signaling pathway

Phosphoinositide 3-kinases or phosphatidylinositol-3-kinases (PI3Ks) belong to a family of enzymes that have serine/threonine kinase activity. These enzymes can be activated by various stimuli including growth factors, antigens, cytokines [157,158], and are capable of phosphorylating the third position hydroxyl group of the inositol ring of phosphatidylinositol (PtdIns) [157,159]. This family is composed of four classes, which differ in their structure and functions (known as Ia, Ib, II, and III). However, all of them contain at least one catalytic domain and one regulatory domain [157,159]. Many PI3K cellular functions rely on the ability of PI3Ks to activate protein kinase B (PKB, also known as Akt) (Figure 1). In humans, three Akt genes have been identified named *akt1*, *akt2*, and *akt3*.

PI3-kinases have been shown to play a major role in diverse cellular functions, including cell growth, proliferation, differentiation, survival, and migration [160-163]. Thus, dysregulation of this pathway may influence different cellular responses that are associated with immunity as well as carcinogenesis (Table 3) [157,164]. It has also been reported that there is a basal activation of the PI3K/Akt pathways in macrophages that is required for their survival [165]. Certain reports have suggested a critical role for PI3K signaling in chronic immune activation by promoting cell survival [166]. For instance, an *in vitro* study has revealed that HIV infection and its protein Tat was sufficient to activate the PI3K/Akt pathway in macrophages [166]. Interestingly, PI3K/Akt inhibitors including Miltefosine, an antiprotozoal drug known to inhibit PI3K/Akt pathway, significantly reduced HIV-1 production from infected macrophages and increased susceptibility to cell death in response to extracellular stress, as compared to uninfected cells [166]. Another study has shown that inhibition of Akt phosphorylation is required for TNF related apoptosis inducing ligand (TRAIL)-induced cell death in HIV infected macrophages [167].

Target Gene	Phenotype
p85$^\alpha$	Decreased B cell development and activation, increased antiviral responses
p85$^\beta$	Increased insulin sensitivity
p110$^\alpha$	Embryonic lethal and defective proliferation
P110$^\beta$	Embryonic lethal
P110$^\gamma$	Decreased T cell development and activation, decreased inflammation, chemotaxis, and oxidative burst
PTEN	Embryonic lethal, autoimmune disease, decreased T cell development, increased T cell activation, and chemotaxis
SHIP1	Increased myeloid cell proliferation and survival, increased B cell activation, chemotaxis, and mast cell degranulation
SHIP2	Perinatal lethal

Table 3. Characteristics of PI3K knockout mice

Viral protein	Effects on M/M	Effects on lymphocytes
gp120	Stimulates STAT1 activation	Stimulates STAT1 activation
p17	Stimulates STAT1 activation	No report
Tat	Stimulates MAPK, Akt activation	Stimulates Akt, MAPK activation
Nef	Stimulates STAT1 & 3, MAPK activation	Stimulates Erk & p38 MAPK activation
Vpr	Stimulates MAPK activation	No report
HIV infection	Inhibits STAT5 activation, Stimulates STAT1, Akt activation	Inhibits STAT5 activation, Stimulates STAT1, MAPK activation

Table 4. HIV viral proteins and their effects on monocytes/macrophages and lymphocytes

4.3.3. MAPK signaling pathway

Mitogen-activated protein kinases (MAPKs) are also a family of enzymes that have serine/threonine kinase activity [168]. This family of kinases is generally activated in response to various extracellular stimuli such as growth factors and inflammatory signals, as well as cellular stress. They regulate different cellular processes including mitosis, proliferation, differentiation, and cell death [168]. The MAPK family is composed of three major subfamilies of kinases known as the extracellular receptor kinases (ERKs), the c-Jun N-terminal kinases/stress-activated protein kinases (JNK/SAPK) and the p38 MAP kinases [169]. Activation of a specific MAP kinase requires activation of a small GTP binding protein (e.g. Ras) which results in the phosphorylation of a series of downstream kinases (Figure 1) [128]. Activation of the MAPK kinase kinase (MAPKKK) (e.g. Raf) leads to the activation of downstream MAPK kinase (MAPKK), and finally, specific MAPK (p38, Erk or JNK) [170,171]. The Erk MAPK family is found in two isoforms called Erk1 and Erk2. Both isoforms are phosphorylated by members of the MEK family, which are often activated by extracellular stimuli such as growth factors, LPS and chemotherapeutic agents [129,172,173]. The JNK family is found in three isoforms named JNK1, JNK2, and JNK3 [174], while the P38 family is found in five different isoforms called p38 (SAPK2), p38β, p38β2, p38γ (SAPK3), and p38δ [175,176]. Both JNK and p38 MAPKs are phosphorylated by SAPK/Erk kinases (SEKs) and mitogen-activated protein kinase kinases (MKKs), which are usually induced by inflammatory cytokines as well as other stressors such as endotoxins, reactive oxygen species, protein synthesis inhibitors, and ultraviolet (UV) irradiation [174,177-179]. MAPKs have been shown to activate various downstream transcription factors such as activator transcription factor (ATF)-2, SP-1 (a member of Specificity Protein/Krüppel-like Factor family) and activator protein (AP)-1, and even STAT3 [178,180-182].

Several reports have shown that activation of the MAPKs resulted in phosphorylation of HIV Rev, Tat, Nef, and p17 proteins and enhanced viral replication [140,183]. Other studies have demonstrated a role for MAPK in regulating monocyte and lymphocyte functions and cell death during HIV infection. For example, in monocytes, it has been shown that the HIV Tat protein stimulates IL-10 production via activation of calcium/MAPK signaling pathways in human monocytes [134,135,184]. Another report has suggested that HIV Vpr is capable of inducing programmed cell death in primary monocytes and the monocytic cell line THP-1 cells [185]. Further, it has been shown that HIV and its protein nef induced FasL, Programmed Death-1 expression and apoptosis in peripheral blood mononuclear cells (PBMCs) and the Jurkat T cell line through activation of the p38 MAPK signaling pathway [138,186].

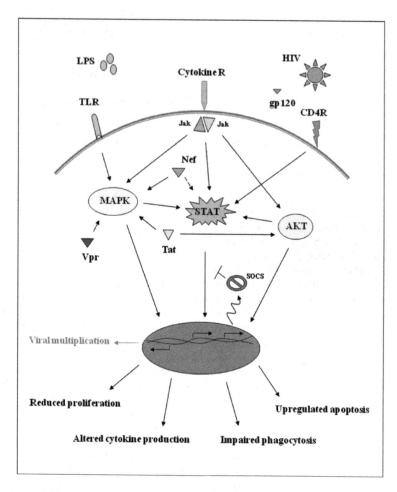

Figure 2. A model for the effect of chronic HIV infection on cellular signal transduction Cell signaling molecules may be regulated directly or indirectly during chronic HIV infection. In the direct setting, HIV and its proteins (Gp120, Nef, Tat, Vpr), through the binding of cellular receptors or internalization by endocytosis, alter signaling pathways including JAK/STAT, PI3K, and MAPK. In the indirect scenario, HIV infection may adversely affects the host cytokine network, which may in turn affect signal transduction. Both scenarios may thus promote viral replication and defective host immune effector functions and reduce immune cell survival [modified from [187].

5. Conclusion

It is well established that HIV targets the immune system and mainly immune cells that express the CD4 surface receptor, but the virus is not exclusive to these cells. Thus, through the course of chronic HIV infection the immune system becomes progressively impaired and unable to protect the body from opportunistic pathogens. This impairment not only includes CD4 T cell depletion, but also the dysregulation of immune cell effector functions, and a skewed cytokine/chemokine expression profile. These effects may be due to the disruption of the described signaling pathways as a result of direct HIV infection, through the action of numerous viral proteins and/or the chronic, but defective state of host immune activation, as summarized in Figure 2. Understanding the molecular mechanisms and identifying the key molecules involved in this impairment may provide important insight towards developing new therapeutic strategies aimed at prolonging the life span of HIV infected individuals and clearing HIV from the host.

Author details

Abdulkarim Alhetheel[1*], Mahmoud Aly[2] and Marko Kryworuchko[3]

*Address all correspondence to: abdulkarimfahad@hotmail.com or aalhetheel@ksu.edu.sa

1 Department of Microbiology, Faculty of Medicine, King Saud University, Riyadh, Saudi Arabia

2 King Abdullah International Medical Research Center, National Guard Hospital, Riyadh, Saudi Arabia

3 Department of Veterinary Microbiology, Western College of Veterinary Medicine, University of Saskatchewan, Saskatoon, Canada

References

[1] Barre-Sinoussi F, Chermann JC, Rey F, Nugeyre MT, Chamaret S, Gruest J, et al. Isolation of a T-lymphotropic retrovirus from a patient at risk for acquired immune deficiency syndrome (AIDS). Science 1983 May 20;220(4599):868-71.

[2] Chinen J, Shearer WT. Molecular virology and immunology of HIV infection. J Allergy Clin Immunol 2002 Aug;110(2):189-98.

[3] Levy JA, Hoffman AD, Kramer SM, Landis JA, Shimabukuro JM, Oshiro LS. Isolation of lymphocytopathic retroviruses from San Francisco patients with AIDS. Science 1984 Aug 24;225(4664):840-2.

[4] Chaplin DD. 1. Overview of the immune response. J Allergy Clin Immunol 2003 Feb; 111(2 Suppl):S442-S459.

[5] Levy JA. Pathogenesis of human immunodeficiency virus infection. Microbiol Rev 1993 Mar;57(1):183-289.

[6] Delves PJ, Roitt IM. The immune system. Second of two parts. N Engl J Med 2000 Jul 13;343(2):108-17.

[7] Delves PJ, Roitt IM. The immune system. First of two parts. N Engl J Med 2000 Jul 6;343(1):37-49.

[8] Medzhitov R, Janeway C, Jr. Innate immunity. N Engl J Med 2000 Aug 3;343(5): 338-44.

[9] Liu YJ. IPC: professional type 1 interferon-producing cells and plasmacytoid dendritic cell precursors. Annu Rev Immunol 2005;23:275-306.

[10] Cullen BR. Is RNA interference involved in intrinsic antiviral immunity in mammals? Nat Immunol 2006 Jun;7(6):563-7.

[11] Uematsu S, Akira S. The role of Toll-like receptors in immune disorders. Expert Opin Biol Ther 2006 Mar;6(3):203-14.

[12] Kato H, Takeuchi O, Sato S, Yoneyama M, Yamamoto M, Matsui K, et al. Differential roles of MDA5 and RIG-I helicases in the recognition of RNA viruses. Nature 2006 May 4;441(7089):101-5.

[13] Hornung V, Guenthner-Biller M, Bourquin C, Ablasser A, Schlee M, Uematsu S, et al. Sequence-specific potent induction of IFN-alpha by short interfering RNA in plasmacytoid dendritic cells through TLR7. Nat Med 2005 Mar;11(3):263-70.

[14] Schlee M, Hornung V, Hartmann G. siRNA and isRNA: two edges of one sword. Mol Ther 2006 Oct;14(4):463-70.

[15] Romagnani S. Regulation of the T cell response. Clin Exp Allergy 2006 Nov;36(11): 1357-66.

[16] Mosmann TR, Coffman RL. TH1 and TH2 cells: different patterns of lymphokine secretion lead to different functional properties. Annu Rev Immunol 1989;7:145-73.

[17] Itoh K, Hirohata S. The role of IL-10 in human B cell activation, proliferation, and differentiation. J Immunol 1995 May 1;154(9):4341-50.

[18] Paul WE. Interleukin-4: a prototypic immunoregulatory lymphokine. Blood 1991 May 1;77(9):1859-70.

[19] de Jong MA, Geijtenbeek TB. Human immunodeficiency virus-1 acquisition in genital mucosa: Langerhans cells as key-players. J Intern Med 2009 Jan;265(1):18-28.

[20] Iqbal SM, Kaul R. Mucosal innate immunity as a determinant of HIV susceptibility. Am J Reprod Immunol 2008 Jan;59(1):44-54.

[21] Sharma D, Bhattacharya J. Cellular & molecular basis of HIV-associated neuropathogenesis. Indian J Med Res 2009 Jun;129(6):637-51.

[22] Boasso A, Shearer GM. Chronic innate immune activation as a cause of HIV-1 immunopathogenesis. Clin Immunol 2008 Mar;126(3):235-42.

[23] Cadogan M, Dalgleish AG. HIV immunopathogenesis and strategies for intervention. Lancet Infect Dis 2008 Nov;8(11):675-84.

[24] Yoo J, Chen H, Kraus T, Hirsch D, Polyak S, George I, et al. Altered cytokine production and accessory cell function after HIV-1 infection. J Immunol 1996 Aug 1;157(3): 1313-20.

[25] Baqui AA, Meiller TF, Zhang M, Falkler WA, Jr. The effects of HIV viral load on the phagocytic activity of monocytes activated with lipopolysaccharide from oral microorganisms. Immunopharmacol Immunotoxicol 1999 Aug;21(3):421-38.

[26] Kedzierska K, Azzam R, Ellery P, Mak J, Jaworowski A, Crowe SM. Defective phagocytosis by human monocyte/macrophages following HIV-1 infection: underlying mechanisms and modulation by adjunctive cytokine therapy. J Clin Virol 2003 Feb; 26(2):247-63.

[27] Thomas CA, Weinberger OK, Ziegler BL, Greenberg S, Schieren I, Silverstein SC, et al. Human immunodeficiency virus-1 env impairs Fc receptor-mediated phagocytosis via a cyclic adenosine monophosphate-dependent mechanism. Blood 1997 Nov 1;90(9):3760-5.

[28] Amirayan-Chevillard N, Tissot-Dupont H, Capo C, Brunet C, Dignat-George F, Obadia Y, et al. Impact of highly active anti-retroviral therapy (HAART) on cytokine production and monocyte subsets in HIV-infected patients. Clin Exp Immunol 2000 Apr; 120(1):107-12.

[29] Choe W, Volsky DJ, Potash MJ. Induction of rapid and extensive beta-chemokine synthesis in macrophages by human immunodeficiency virus type 1 and gp120, independently of their coreceptor phenotype. J Virol 2001 Nov;75(22):10738-45.

[30] Denis M, Ghadirian E. Alveolar macrophages from subjects infected with HIV-1 express macrophage inflammatory protein-1 alpha (MIP-1 alpha): contribution to the CD8+ alveolitis. Clin Exp Immunol 1994 May;96(2):187-92.

[31] Tartakovsky B, Turner D, Vardinon N, Burke M, Yust I. Increased intracellular accumulation of macrophage inflammatory protein 1beta and its decreased secretion correlate with advanced HIV disease. J Acquir Immune Defic Syndr Hum Retrovirol 1999 Apr 15;20(5):420-2.

[32] Polyak S, Chen H, Hirsch D, George I, Hershberg R, Sperber K. Impaired class II expression and antigen uptake in monocytic cells after HIV-1 infection. J Immunol 1997 Sep 1;159(5):2177-88.

[33] Shao L, Sperber K. Impaired regulation of HLA-DR expression in human immunodeficiency virus-infected monocytes. Clin Diagn Lab Immunol 2002 Jul;9(4):739-46.

[34] Clerici M, Hakim FT, Venzon DJ, Blatt S, Hendrix CW, Wynn TA, et al. Changes in interleukin-2 and interleukin-4 production in asymptomatic, human immunodeficiency virus-seropositive individuals. J Clin Invest 1993 Mar;91(3):759-65.

[35] Clerici M, Shearer GM. A TH1-->TH2 switch is a critical step in the etiology of HIV infection. Immunol Today 1993 Mar;14(3):107-11.

[36] Sirskyj D, Theze J, Kumar A, Kryworuchko M. Disruption of the gamma c cytokine network in T cells during HIV infection. Cytokine 2008 Jul;43(1):1-14.

[37] Kryworuchko M, Pasquier V, Theze J. Human immunodeficiency virus-1 envelope glycoproteins and anti-CD4 antibodies inhibit interleukin-2-induced Jak/STAT signalling in human CD4 T lymphocytes. Clin Exp Immunol 2003 Mar;131(3):422-7.

[38] Kryworuchko M, Pasquier V, Keller H, David D, Goujard C, Gilquin J, et al. Defective interleukin-2-dependent STAT5 signalling in CD8 T lymphocytes from HIV-positive patients: restoration by antiretroviral therapy. AIDS 2004 Feb 20;18(3):421-6.

[39] Alhetheel A, Yakubtsov Y, Abdkader K, Sant N, az-Mitoma F, Kumar A, et al. Amplification of the signal transducer and activator of transcription I signaling pathway and its association with apoptosis in monocytes from HIV-infected patients. AIDS 2008 Jun 19;22(10):1137-44.

[40] Benoit A, Abdkader K, Sirskyj D, Alhetheel A, Sant N, az-Mitoma F, et al. Inverse association of repressor growth factor independent-1 with CD8 T cell interleukin (IL)-7 receptor [alpha] expression and limited signal transducers and activators of transcription signaling in response to IL-7 among [gamma]-chain cytokines in HIV patients. AIDS 2009 Jul 17;23(11):1341-7.

[41] Vranjkovic A, Crawley AM, Patey A, Angel JB. IL-7-dependent STAT-5 activation and CD8+ T cell proliferation are impaired in HIV infection. J Leukoc Biol 2011 Apr; 89(4):499-506.

[42] Hardy GA, Sieg SF, Rodriguez B, Jiang W, Asaad R, Lederman MM, et al. Desensitization to type I interferon in HIV-1 infection correlates with markers of immune activation and disease progression. Blood 2009 May 28;113(22):5497-505.

[43] Westendorp MO, Frank R, Ochsenbauer C, Stricker K, Dhein J, Walczak H, et al. Sensitization of T cells to CD95-mediated apoptosis by HIV-1 Tat and gp120. Nature 1995 Jun 8;375(6531):497-500.

[44] Yang Y, Tikhonov I, Ruckwardt TJ, Djavani M, Zapata JC, Pauza CD, et al. Monocytes treated with human immunodeficiency virus Tat kill uninfected CD4(+) cells by a tumor necrosis factor-related apoptosis-induced ligand-mediated mechanism. J Virol 2003 Jun;77(12):6700-8.

[45] Zhang M, Li X, Pang X, Ding L, Wood O, Clouse K, et al. Identification of a potential HIV-induced source of bystander-mediated apoptosis in T cells: upregulation of trail in primary human macrophages by HIV-1 tat. J Biomed Sci 2001 May;8(3):290-6.

[46] Zhou D, Spector SA. Human immunodeficiency virus type-1 infection inhibits autophagy. AIDS 2008 Mar 30;22(6):695-9.

[47] Jang HR, Rabb H. The innate immune response in ischemic acute kidney injury. Clin Immunol 2009 Jan;130(1):41-50.

[48] Nadeen Ikram, Khalid Hassan, Samina Tufail. Cytokines. Int J Pathology 2004;2(1): 47-58.

[49] Aman MJ, Leonard WJ. Cytokine signaling: cytokine-inducible signaling inhibitors. Curr Biol 1997 Dec 1;7(12):R784-R788.

[50] Cohen MC, Cohen S. Cytokine function: a study in biologic diversity. Am J Clin Pathol 1996 May;105(5):589-98.

[51] Mueller SN, Hosiawa-Meagher KA, Konieczny BT, Sullivan BM, Bachmann MF, Locksley RM, et al. Regulation of homeostatic chemokine expression and cell trafficking during immune responses. Science 2007 Aug 3;317(5838):670-4.

[52] Lucey DR, Clerici M, Shearer GM. Type 1 and type 2 cytokine dysregulation in human infectious, neoplastic, and inflammatory diseases. Clin Microbiol Rev 1996 Oct; 9(4):532-62.

[53] Alfano M, Poli G. The cytokine network in HIV infection. Curr Mol Med 2002 Dec; 2(8):677-89.

[54] Clerici M, Sarin A, Coffman RL, Wynn TA, Blatt SP, Hendrix CW, et al. Type 1/type 2 cytokine modulation of T-cell programmed cell death as a model for human immunodeficiency virus pathogenesis. Proc Natl Acad Sci U S A 1994 Dec 6;91(25):11811-5.

[55] Estaquier J, Ameisen JC. A role for T-helper type-1 and type-2 cytokines in the regulation of human monocyte apoptosis. Blood 1997 Aug 15;90(4):1618-25.

[56] Sinicco A, Biglino A, Sciandra M, Forno B, Pollono AM, Raiteri R, et al. Cytokine network and acute primary HIV-1 infection. AIDS 1993 Sep;7(9):1167-72.

[57] Schroder K, Hertzog PJ, Ravasi T, Hume DA. Interferon-gamma: an overview of signals, mechanisms and functions. J Leukoc Biol 2004 Feb;75(2):163-89.

[58] Stark GR, Kerr IM, Williams BR, Silverman RH, Schreiber RD. How cells respond to interferons. Annu Rev Biochem 1998;67:227-64.

[59] Barrionuevo P, Beigier-Bompadre M, De La BS, Alves-Rosa MF, Fernandez G, Palermo MS, et al. Immune complexes (IC) down-regulate the basal and interferon-gamma-induced expression of MHC class II on human monocytes. Clin Exp Immunol 2001 Aug;125(2):251-7.

[60] Dellacasagrande J, Ghigo E, Raoult D, Capo C, Mege JL. IFN-gamma-induced apoptosis and microbicidal activity in monocytes harboring the intracellular bacterium Coxiella burnetii require membrane TNF and homotypic cell adherence. J Immunol 2002 Dec 1;169(11):6309-15.

[61] Kedzierska K, Paukovics G, Handley A, Hewish M, Hocking J, Cameron PU, et al. Interferon-gamma therapy activates human monocytes for enhanced phagocytosis of Mycobacterium avium complex in HIV-infected individuals. HIV Clin Trials 2004 Mar;5(2):80-5.

[62] Lehn M, Weiser WY, Engelhorn S, Gillis S, Remold HG. IL-4 inhibits H2O2 production and antileishmanial capacity of human cultured monocytes mediated by IFN-gamma. J Immunol 1989 Nov 1;143(9):3020-4.

[63] Griffith TS, Wiley SR, Kubin MZ, Sedger LM, Maliszewski CR, Fanger NA. Monocyte-mediated tumoricidal activity via the tumor necrosis factor-related cytokine, TRAIL. J Exp Med 1999 Apr 19;189(8):1343-54.

[64] Harris J, De Haro SA, Master SS, Keane J, Roberts EA, Delgado M, et al. T helper 2 cytokines inhibit autophagic control of intracellular Mycobacterium tuberculosis. Immunity 2007 Sep;27(3):505-17.

[65] Gavrilescu LC, Butcher BA, Del Rio L, Taylor GA, Denkers EY. STAT1 is essential for antimicrobial effector function but dispensable for gamma interferon production during Toxoplasma gondii infection. Infect Immun 2004 Mar;72(3):1257-64.

[66] Dalton DK, Pitts-Meek S, Keshav S, Figari IS, Bradley A, Stewart TA. Multiple defects of immune cell function in mice with disrupted interferon-gamma genes. Science 1993 Mar 19;259(5102):1739-42.

[67] Durbin JE, Hackenmiller R, Simon MC, Levy DE. Targeted disruption of the mouse Stat1 gene results in compromised innate immunity to viral disease. Cell 1996 Feb 9;84(3):443-50.

[68] Huang S, Hendriks W, Althage A, Hemmi S, Bluethmann H, Kamijo R, et al. Immune response in mice that lack the interferon-gamma receptor. Science 1993 Mar 19;259(5102):1742-5.

[69] Jouanguy E, Altare F, Lamhamedi-Cherradi S, Casanova JL. Infections in IFNGR-1-deficient children. J Interferon Cytokine Res 1997 Oct;17(10):583-7.

[70] Meraz MA, White JM, Sheehan KC, Bach EA, Rodig SJ, Dighe AS, et al. Targeted disruption of the Stat1 gene in mice reveals unexpected physiologic specificity in the JAK-STAT signaling pathway. Cell 1996 Feb 9;84(3):431-42.

[71] Armitage JO. Emerging applications of recombinant human granulocyte-macrophage colony-stimulating factor. Blood 1998 Dec 15;92(12):4491-508.

[72] Hamilton JA, Anderson GP. GM-CSF Biology. Growth Factors 2004 Dec;22(4):225-31.

[73] Moore KW, O'Garra A, de Waal MR, Vieira P, Mosmann TR. Interleukin-10. Annu Rev Immunol 1993;11:165-90.

[74] Moore KW, de Waal MR, Coffman RL, O'Garra A. Interleukin-10 and the interleukin-10 receptor. Annu Rev Immunol 2001;19:683-765.

[75] Akdis CA, Blaser K. Mechanisms of interleukin-10-mediated immune suppression. Immunology 2001 Jun;103(2):131-6.

[76] Redpath S, Ghazal P, Gascoigne NR. Hijacking and exploitation of IL-10 by intracellular pathogens. Trends Microbiol 2001 Feb;9(2):86-92.

[77] Cenci E, Romani L, Mencacci A, Spaccapelo R, Schiaffella E, Puccetti P, et al. Interleukin-4 and interleukin-10 inhibit nitric oxide-dependent macrophage killing of Candida albicans. Eur J Immunol 1993 May;23(5):1034-8.

[78] Levy Y, Brouet JC. Interleukin-10 prevents spontaneous death of germinal center B cells by induction of the bcl-2 protein. J Clin Invest 1994 Jan;93(1):424-8.

[79] Crawford RM, Finbloom DS, Ohara J, Paul WE, Meltzer MS. B cell stimulatory factor-1 (interleukin 4) activates macrophages for increased tumoricidal activity and expression of Ia antigens. J Immunol 1987 Jul 1;139(1):135-41.

[80] Littman BH, Dastvan FF, Carlson PL, Sanders KM. Regulation of monocyte/macrophage C2 production and HLA-DR expression by IL-4 (BSF-1) and IFN-gamma. J Immunol 1989 Jan 15;142(2):520-5.

[81] Raveh D, Kruskal BA, Farland J, Ezekowitz RA. Th1 and Th2 cytokines cooperate to stimulate mannose-receptor-mediated phagocytosis. J Leukoc Biol 1998 Jul;64(1): 108-13.

[82] Stein M, Keshav S, Harris N, Gordon S. Interleukin 4 potently enhances murine macrophage mannose receptor activity: a marker of alternative immunologic macrophage activation. J Exp Med 1992 Jul 1;176(1):287-92.

[83] te Velde AA, Klomp JP, Yard BA, de Vries JE, Figdor CG. Modulation of phenotypic and functional properties of human peripheral blood monocytes by IL-4. J Immunol 1988 Mar 1;140(5):1548-54.

[84] Vercelli D, Jabara HH, Lee BW, Woodland N, Geha RS, Leung DY. Human recombinant interleukin 4 induces Fc epsilon R2/CD23 on normal human monocytes. J Exp Med 1988 Apr 1;167(4):1406-16.

[85] Cheung DL, Hart PH, Vitti GF, Whitty GA, Hamilton JA. Contrasting effects of interferon-gamma and interleukin-4 on the interleukin-6 activity of stimulated human monocytes. Immunology 1990 Sep;71(1):70-5.

[86] Donnelly RP, Fenton MJ, Kaufman JD, Gerrard TL. IL-1 expression in human monocytes is transcriptionally and posttranscriptionally regulated by IL-4. J Immunol 1991 May 15;146(10):3431-6.

[87] Hamilton JA, Whitty GA, Royston AK, Cebon J, Layton JE. Interleukin-4 suppresses granulocyte colony-stimulating factor and granulocyte-macrophage colony-stimulating factor levels in stimulated human monocytes. Immunology 1992 Aug;76(4): 566-71.

[88] Hart PH, Jones CA, Finlay-Jones JJ. Interleukin-4 suppression of monocyte tumour necrosis factor-alpha production. Dependence on protein synthesis but not on cyclic AMP production. Immunology 1992 Aug;76(4):560-5.

[89] Lee JD, Swisher SG, Minehart EH, McBride WH, Economou JS. Interleukin-4 down-regulates interleukin-6 production in human peripheral blood mononuclear cells. J Leukoc Biol 1990 May;47(5):475-9.

[90] Standiford TJ, Strieter RM, Chensue SW, Westwick J, Kasahara K, Kunkel SL. IL-4 inhibits the expression of IL-8 from stimulated human monocytes. J Immunol 1990 Sep 1;145(5):1435-9.

[91] te Velde AA, Huijbens RJ, Heije K, de Vries JE, Figdor CG. Interleukin-4 (IL-4) inhibits secretion of IL-1 beta, tumor necrosis factor alpha, and IL-6 by human monocytes. Blood 1990 Oct 1;76(7):1392-7.

[92] Weiss L, Haeffner-Cavaillon N, Laude M, Cavaillon JM, Kazatchkine MD. Human T cells and interleukin 4 inhibit the release of interleukin 1 induced by lipopolysaccharide in serum-free cultures of autologous monocytes. Eur J Immunol 1989 Jul;19(7): 1347-50.

[93] Wong HL, Lotze MT, Wahl LM, Wahl SM. Administration of recombinant IL-4 to humans regulates gene expression, phenotype, and function in circulating monocytes. J Immunol 1992 Apr 1;148(7):2118-25.

[94] Yanagawa H, Sone S, Sugihara K, Tanaka K, Ogura T. Interleukin-4 downregulates interleukin-6 production by human alveolar macrophages at protein and mRNA levels. Microbiol Immunol 1991;35(10):879-93.

[95] Ho JL, He SH, Rios MJ, Wick EA. Interleukin-4 inhibits human macrophage activation by tumor necrosis factor, granulocyte-monocyte colony-stimulating factor, and interleukin-3 for antileishmanial activity and oxidative burst capacity. J Infect Dis 1992 Feb;165(2):344-51.

[96] Elliott MJ, Gamble JR, Park LS, Vadas MA, Lopez AF. Inhibition of human monocyte adhesion by interleukin-4. Blood 1991 Jun 15;77(12):2739-45.

[97] Lauener RP, Goyert SM, Geha RS, Vercelli D. Interleukin 4 down-regulates the expression of CD14 in normal human monocytes. Eur J Immunol 1990 Nov;20(11): 2375-81.

[98] Hudson MM, Markowitz AB, Gutterman JU, Knowles RD, Snyder JS, Kleinerman ES. Effect of recombinant human interleukin 4 on human monocyte activity. Cancer Res 1990 Jun 1;50(11):3154-8.

[99]   Leone A, Picker LJ, Sodora DL. IL-2, IL-7 and IL-15 as immuno-modulators during SIV/HIV vaccination and treatment. Curr HIV Res 2009 Jan;7(1):83-90.

[100] Refaeli Y, Van PL, London CA, Tschopp J, Abbas AK. Biochemical mechanisms of IL-2-regulated Fas-mediated T cell apoptosis. Immunity 1998 May;8(5):615-23.

[101] Van PL, Abbas AK. Homeostasis and self-tolerance in the immune system: turning lymphocytes off. Science 1998 Apr 10;280(5361):243-8.

[102] Durum SK, Candeias S, Nakajima H, Leonard WJ, Baird AM, Berg LJ, et al. Interleukin 7 receptor control of T cell receptor gamma gene rearrangement: role of receptor-associated chains and locus accessibility. J Exp Med 1998 Dec 21;188(12):2233-41.

[103] Hare KJ, Jenkinson EJ, Anderson G. An essential role for the IL-7 receptor during intrathymic expansion of the positively selected neonatal T cell repertoire. J Immunol 2000 Sep 1;165(5):2410-4.

[104] Huang J, Muegge K. Control of chromatin accessibility for V(D)J recombination by interleukin-7. J Leukoc Biol 2001 Jun;69(6):907-11.

[105] Kang J, DiBenedetto B, Narayan K, Zhao H, Der SD, Chambers CA. STAT5 is required for thymopoiesis in a development stage-specific manner. J Immunol 2004 Aug 15;173(4):2307-14.

[106] Diallo M, Zheng Y, Chen X, He Y, Zhou H, Chen Z. Prospect of IL-2, IL-7, IL-15 and IL-21 for HIV immune-based therapy. Zhong Nan Da Xue Xue Bao Yi Xue Ban 2011 Nov;36(11):1037-45.

[107] Ameglio F, Cordiali FP, Solmone M, Bonifati C, Prignano G, Giglio A, et al. Serum IL-10 levels in HIV-positive subjects: correlation with CDC stages. J Biol Regul Homeost Agents 1994 Apr;8(2):48-52.

[108] Minagawa T, Mizuno K, Hirano S, Asano M, Numata A, Kohanawa M, et al. Detection of high levels of immunoreactive human beta-1 interferon in sera from HIV-infected patients. Life Sci 1989;45(11):iii-vii.

[109] Orsilles MA, Pieri E, Cooke P, Caula C. IL-2 and IL-10 serum levels in HIV-1-infected patients with or without active antiretroviral therapy. APMIS 2006 Jan;114(1):55-60.

[110] Pugliese A, Torre D, Saini A, Pagliano G, Gallo G, Pistono PG, et al. Cytokine detection in HIV-1/HHV-8 co-infected subjects. Cell Biochem Funct 2002 Sep;20(3):191-4.

[111] Reddy MM, Sorrell SJ, Lange M, Grieco MH. Tumor necrosis factor and HIV P24 antigen levels in serum of HIV-infected populations. J Acquir Immune Defic Syndr 1988;1(5):436-40.

[112] Sato A, Tsuji K, Yamamura M, Morita Y, Kanzaki H, Tada J, et al. Increased type 2 cytokine expression by both CD4+ CD45RO+ T cells and CD8+ CD45RO+ T cells in blood circulation is associated with high serum IgE but not with atopic dermatitis. J Invest Dermatol 1998 Dec;111(6):1079-84.

[113] Sindhu S, Toma E, Cordeiro P, Ahmad R, Morisset R, Menezes J. Relationship of in vivo and ex vivo levels of TH1 and TH2 cytokines with viremia in HAART patients with and without opportunistic infections. J Med Virol 2006 Apr;78(4):431-9.

[114] Srikanth P, Castillo RC, Sridharan G, John TJ, Zachariah A, Mathai D, et al. Increase in plasma IL-10 levels and rapid loss of CD4+ T cells among HIV-infected individuals in south India. Int J STD AIDS 2000 Jan;11(1):49-51.

[115] Stylianou E, Aukrust P, Kvale D, Muller F, Froland SS. IL-10 in HIV infection: increasing serum IL-10 levels with disease progression--down-regulatory effect of potent anti-retroviral therapy. Clin Exp Immunol 1999 Apr;116(1):115-20.

[116] de GM, Castrillo JM, Fernandez Guerrero ML. Visceral leishmaniasis in patients with AIDS: report of three cases treated with pentavalent antimony and interferon-gamma. Clin Infect Dis 1993 Jul;17(1):56-8.

[117] Squires KE, Brown ST, Armstrong D, Murphy WF, Murray HW. Interferon-gamma treatment for Mycobacterium avium-intracellular complex bacillemia in patients with AIDS. J Infect Dis 1992 Sep;166(3):686-7.

[118] Sabbatini F, Bandera A, Ferrario G, Trabattoni D, Marchetti G, Franzetti F, et al. Qualitative immune modulation by interleukin-2 (IL-2) adjuvant therapy in immunological non responder HIV-infected patients. PLoS One 2010;5(11):e14119.

[119] Ihle JN. The Stat family in cytokine signaling. Curr Opin Cell Biol 2001 Apr;13(2): 211-7.

[120] Imada K, Leonard WJ. The Jak-STAT pathway. Mol Immunol 2000 Jan;37(1-2):1-11.

[121] Levy DE, Darnell JE, Jr. Stats: transcriptional control and biological impact. Nat Rev Mol Cell Biol 2002 Sep;3(9):651-62.

[122] O'Shea JJ. Jaks, STATs, cytokine signal transduction, and immunoregulation: are we there yet? Immunity 1997 Jul;7(1):1-11.

[123] Ward AC, Touw I, Yoshimura A. The Jak-Stat pathway in normal and perturbed hematopoiesis. Blood 2000 Jan 1;95(1):19-29.

[124] Pokrovskaja K, Panaretakis T, Grander D. Alternative signaling pathways regulating type I interferon-induced apoptosis. J Interferon Cytokine Res 2005 Dec;25(12): 799-810.

[125] Rani MR, Ransohoff RM. Alternative and accessory pathways in the regulation of IFN-beta-mediated gene expression. J Interferon Cytokine Res 2005 Dec;25(12): 788-98.

[126] Wong CK, Zhang J, Ip WK, Lam CW. Intracellular signal transduction in eosinophils and its clinical significance. Immunopharmacol Immunotoxicol 2002 May;24(2): 165-86.

[127] Kolch W. Meaningful relationships: the regulation of the Ras/Raf/MEK/ERK pathway by protein interactions. Biochem J 2000 Oct 15;351 Pt 2:289-305.

[128] Scita G, Tenca P, Frittoli E, Tocchetti A, Innocenti M, Giardina G, et al. Signaling from Ras to Rac and beyond: not just a matter of GEFs. EMBO J 2000 Jun 1;19(11): 2393-8.

[129] Caunt CJ, Finch AR, Sedgley KR, McArdle CA. Seven-transmembrane receptor signalling and ERK compartmentalization. Trends Endocrinol Metab 2006 Sep;17(7): 276-83.

[130] Darnell JE, Jr., Kerr IM, Stark GR. Jak-STAT pathways and transcriptional activation in response to IFNs and other extracellular signaling proteins. Science 1994 Jun 3;264(5164):1415-21.

[131] Stepkowski SM, Kirken RA. Janus tyrosine kinases and signal transducers and activators of transcription regulate critical functions of T cells in allograft rejection and transplantation tolerance. Transplantation 2006 Aug 15;82(3):295-303.

[132] Jin H, Lanning NJ, Carter-Su C. JAK2, but not Src family kinases, is required for STAT, ERK, and Akt signaling in response to growth hormone in preadipocytes and hepatoma cells. Mol Endocrinol 2008 Aug;22(8):1825-41.

[133] Nguyen H, Ramana CV, Bayes J, Stark GR. Roles of phosphatidylinositol 3-kinase in interferon-gamma-dependent phosphorylation of STAT1 on serine 727 and activation of gene expression. J Biol Chem 2001 Sep 7;276(36):33361-8.

[134] Gee K, Angel JB, Ma W, Mishra S, Gajanayaka N, Parato K, et al. Intracellular HIV-Tat expression induces IL-10 synthesis by the CREB-1 transcription factor through Ser133 phosphorylation and its regulation by the ERK1/2 MAPK in human monocytic cells. J Biol Chem 2006 Oct 20;281(42):31647-58.

[135] Leghmari K, Bennasser Y, Tkaczuk J, Bahraoui E. HIV-1 Tat protein induces IL-10 production by an alternative TNF-alpha-independent pathway in monocytes: role of PKC-delta and p38 MAP kinase. Cell Immunol 2008 May;253(1-2):45-53.

[136] Mischiati C, Pironi F, Milani D, Giacca M, Mirandola P, Capitani S, et al. Extracellular HIV-1 Tat protein differentially activates the JNK and ERK/MAPK pathways in CD4 T cells. AIDS 1999 Sep 10;13(13):1637-45.

[137] Mishra S, Mishra JP, Kumar A. Activation of JNK-dependent pathway is required for HIV viral protein R-induced apoptosis in human monocytic cells: involvement of antiapoptotic BCL2 and c-IAP1 genes. J Biol Chem 2007 Feb 16;282(7):4288-300.

[138] Muthumani K, Choo AY, Hwang DS, Premkumar A, Dayes NS, Harris C, et al. HIV-1 Nef-induced FasL induction and bystander killing requires p38 MAPK activation. Blood 2005 Sep 15;106(6):2059-68.

[139] Renga B, Francisci D, D'Amore C, Schiaroli E, Mencarelli A, Cipriani S, et al. The HIV matrix protein p17 subverts nuclear receptors expression and induces a STAT1-dependent proinflammatory phenotype in monocytes. PLoS One 2012;7(4):e35924.

[140] Yang X, Gabuzda D. Regulation of human immunodeficiency virus type 1 infectivity by the ERK mitogen-activated protein kinase signaling pathway. J Virol 1999 Apr; 73(4):3460-6.

[141] Federico M, Percario Z, Olivetta E, Fiorucci G, Muratori C, Micheli A, et al. HIV-1 Nef activates STAT1 in human monocytes/macrophages through the release of soluble factors. Blood 2001 Nov 1;98(9):2752-61.

[142] Kohler JJ, Tuttle DL, Coberley CR, Sleasman JW, Goodenow MM. Human immunodeficiency virus type 1 (HIV-1) induces activation of multiple STATs in CD4+ cells of lymphocyte or monocyte/macrophage lineages. J Leukoc Biol 2003 Mar;73(3):407-16.

[143] Percario Z, Olivetta E, Fiorucci G, Mangino G, Peretti S, Romeo G, et al. Human immunodeficiency virus type 1 (HIV-1) Nef activates STAT3 in primary human monocyte/macrophages through the release of soluble factors: involvement of Nef domains interacting with the cell endocytotic machinery. J Leukoc Biol 2003 Nov; 74(5):821-32.

[144] Selliah N, Finkel TH. HIV-1 NL4-3, but not IIIB, inhibits JAK3/STAT5 activation in CD4(+) T cells. Virology 2001 Aug 1;286(2):412-21.

[145] Vyakarnam A, Matear P, Meager A, Kelly G, Stanley B, Weller I, et al. Altered production of tumour necrosis factors alpha and beta and interferon gamma by HIV-infected individuals. Clin Exp Immunol 1991 Apr;84(1):109-15.

[146] Herbein G, Gras G, Khan KA, Abbas W. Macrophage signaling in HIV-1 infection. Retrovirology 2010;7:34.

[147] Bromberg J, Darnell JE, Jr. The role of STATs in transcriptional control and their impact on cellular function. Oncogene 2000 May 15;19(21):2468-73.

[148] Calo V, Migliavacca M, Bazan V, Macaluso M, Buscemi M, Gebbia N, et al. STAT proteins: from normal control of cellular events to tumorigenesis. J Cell Physiol 2003 Nov;197(2):157-68.

[149] Hebenstreit D, Horejs-Hoeck J, Duschl A. JAK/STAT-dependent gene regulation by cytokines. Drug News Perspect 2005 May;18(4):243-9.

[150] Bach EA, Aguet M, Schreiber RD. The IFN gamma receptor: a paradigm for cytokine receptor signaling. Annu Rev Immunol 1997;15:563-91.

[151] Darnell JE, Jr. STATs and gene regulation. Science 1997 Sep 12;277(5332):1630-5.

[152] Lehtonen A, Matikainen S, Julkunen I. Interferons up-regulate STAT1, STAT2, and IRF family transcription factor gene expression in human peripheral blood mononuclear cells and macrophages. J Immunol 1997 Jul 15;159(2):794-803.

[153] Lehtonen A, Matikainen S, Miettinen M, Julkunen I. Granulocyte-macrophage colony-stimulating factor (GM-CSF)-induced STAT5 activation and target-gene expression during human monocyte/macrophage differentiation. J Leukoc Biol 2002 Mar; 71(3):511-9.

[154] Kohlhuber F, Rogers NC, Watling D, Feng J, Guschin D, Briscoe J, et al. A JAK1/JAK2 chimera can sustain alpha and gamma interferon responses. Mol Cell Biol 1997 Feb; 17(2):695-706.

[155] Bovolenta C, Lorini AL, Mantelli B, Camorali L, Novelli F, Biswas P, et al. A selective defect of IFN-gamma- but not of IFN-alpha-induced JAK/STAT pathway in a subset of U937 clones prevents the antiretroviral effect of IFN-gamma against HIV-1. J Immunol 1999 Jan 1;162(1):323-30.

[156] Warby TJ, Crowe SM, Jaworowski A. Human immunodeficiency virus type 1 infection inhibits granulocyte-macrophage colony-stimulating factor-induced activation of STAT5A in human monocyte-derived macrophages. J Virol 2003 Dec;77(23): 12630-8.

[157] Fruman DA, Meyers RE, Cantley LC. Phosphoinositide kinases. Annu Rev Biochem 1998;67:481-507.

[158] Rodriguez-Viciana P, Warne PH, Dhand R, Vanhaesebroeck B, Gout I, Fry MJ, et al. Phosphatidylinositol-3-OH kinase as a direct target of Ras. Nature 1994 Aug 18;370(6490):527-32.

[159] Wymann MP, Pirola L. Structure and function of phosphoinositide 3-kinases. Biochim Biophys Acta 1998 Dec 8;1436(1-2):127-50.

[160] Katso R, Okkenhaug K, Ahmadi K, White S, Timms J, Waterfield MD. Cellular function of phosphoinositide 3-kinases: implications for development, homeostasis, and cancer. Annu Rev Cell Dev Biol 2001;17:615-75.

[161] Koyasu S. The role of PI3K in immune cells. Nat Immunol 2003 Apr;4(4):313-9.

[162] Vanhaesebroeck B, Leevers SJ, Ahmadi K, Timms J, Katso R, Driscoll PC, et al. Synthesis and function of 3-phosphorylated inositol lipids. Annu Rev Biochem 2001;70:535-602.

[163] Deane JA, Fruman DA. Phosphoinositide 3-kinase: diverse roles in immune cell activation. Annu Rev Immunol 2004;22:563-98.

[164] Sasaki T, Suzuki A, Sasaki J, Penninger JM. Phosphoinositide 3-kinases in immunity: lessons from knockout mice. J Biochem 2002 Apr;131(4):495-501.

[165] Liu H, Perlman H, Pagliari LJ, Pope RM. Constitutively activated Akt-1 is vital for the survival of human monocyte-differentiated macrophages. Role of Mcl-1, independent of nuclear factor (NF)-kappaB, Bad, or caspase activation. J Exp Med 2001 Jul 16;194(2):113-26.

[166] Chugh P, Bradel-Tretheway B, Monteiro-Filho CM, Planelles V, Maggirwar SB, Dewhurst S, et al. Akt inhibitors as an HIV-1 infected macrophage-specific anti-viral therapy. Retrovirology 2008;5:11.

[167] Huang Y, Erdmann N, Peng H, Herek S, Davis JS, Luo X, et al. TRAIL-mediated apoptosis in HIV-1-infected macrophages is dependent on the inhibition of Akt-1 phosphorylation. J Immunol 2006 Aug 15;177(4):2304-13.

[168] Cowan KJ, Storey KB. Mitogen-activated protein kinases: new signaling pathways functioning in cellular responses to environmental stress. J Exp Biol 2003 Apr;206(Pt 7):1107-15.

[169] Zhang YL, Dong C. MAP kinases in immune responses. Cell Mol Immunol 2005 Feb; 2(1):20-7.

[170] Dong C, Davis RJ, Flavell RA. Signaling by the JNK group of MAP kinases. c-jun N-terminal Kinase. J Clin Immunol 2001 Jul;21(4):253-7.

[171] Dong C, Davis RJ, Flavell RA. MAP kinases in the immune response. Annu Rev Immunol 2002;20:55-72.

[172] Nishimoto S, Nishida E. MAPK signalling: ERK5 versus ERK1/2. EMBO Rep 2006 Aug;7(8):782-6.

[173] Sugden PH, Clerk A. Regulation of the ERK subgroup of MAP kinase cascades through G protein-coupled receptors. Cell Signal 1997 Aug;9(5):337-51.

[174] Gupta S, Barrett T, Whitmarsh AJ, Cavanagh J, Sluss HK, Derijard B, et al. Selective interaction of JNK protein kinase isoforms with transcription factors. EMBO J 1996 Jun 3;15(11):2760-70.

[175] Hale KK, Trollinger D, Rihanek M, Manthey CL. Differential expression and activation of p38 mitogen-activated protein kinase alpha, beta, gamma, and delta in inflammatory cell lineages. J Immunol 1999 Apr 1;162(7):4246-52.

[176] Ono K, Han J. The p38 signal transduction pathway: activation and function. Cell Signal 2000 Jan;12(1):1-13.

[177] Ashwell JD. The many paths to p38 mitogen-activated protein kinase activation in the immune system. Nat Rev Immunol 2006 Jul;6(7):532-40.

[178] Kyriakis JM, Banerjee P, Nikolakaki E, Dai T, Rubie EA, Ahmad MF, et al. The stress-activated protein kinase subfamily of c-Jun kinases. Nature 1994 May 12;369(6476): 156-60.

[179] Rouse J, Cohen P, Trigon S, Morange M, onso-Llamazares A, Zamanillo D, et al. A novel kinase cascade triggered by stress and heat shock that stimulates MAPKAP kinase-2 and phosphorylation of the small heat shock proteins. Cell 1994 Sep 23;78(6):1027-37.

[180] Chung J, Uchida E, Grammer TC, Blenis J. STAT3 serine phosphorylation by ERK-dependent and -independent pathways negatively modulates its tyrosine phosphorylation. Mol Cell Biol 1997 Nov;17(11):6508-16.

[181] Hibi M, Lin A, Smeal T, Minden A, Karin M. Identification of an oncoprotein- and UV-responsive protein kinase that binds and potentiates the c-Jun activation domain. Genes Dev 1993 Nov;7(11):2135-48.

[182] Zhang S, Liu H, Liu J, Tse CA, Dragunow M, Cooper GJ. Activation of activating transcription factor 2 by p38 MAP kinase during apoptosis induced by human amylin in cultured pancreatic beta-cells. FEBS J 2006 Aug;273(16):3779-91.

[183] Evans P, Sacan A, Ungar L, Tozeren A. Sequence alignment reveals possible MAPK docking motifs on HIV proteins. PLoS One 2010;5(1):e8942.

[184] Gee K, Angel JB, Mishra S, Blahoianu MA, Kumar A. IL-10 regulation by HIV-Tat in primary human monocytic cells: involvement of calmodulin/calmodulin-dependent protein kinase-activated p38 MAPK and Sp-1 and CREB-1 transcription factors. J Immunol 2007 Jan 15;178(2):798-807.

[185] Saxena M, Busca A, Pandey S, Kryworuchko M, Kumar A. CpG protects human monocytic cells against HIV-Vpr-induced apoptosis by cellular inhibitor of apoptosis-2 through the calcium-activated JNK pathway in a TLR9-independent manner. J Immunol 2011 Dec 1;187(11):5865-78.

[186] Muthumani K, Choo AY, Shedlock DJ, Laddy DJ, Sundaram SG, Hirao L, et al. Human immunodeficiency virus type 1 Nef induces programmed death 1 expression through a p38 mitogen-activated protein kinase-dependent mechanism. J Virol 2008 Dec;82(23):11536-44.

[187] Alhetheel A. HIV-induced dysregulation of IFN-gamma signaling and programmed cell death in human primary monocytes. Ph D Thesis, 2010.

Chapter 3

Hematopoietic Stem Cell Transplantation in HIV Infected Patients

Nitya Nathwani

Additional information is available at the end of the chapter

1. Introduction

In the highly active antiretroviral therapy (HAART) era, the survival of HIV infected patients has improved. Opportunistic infections and AIDS related syndromes in these individuals have declined (Palella et al, 1998). HIV infected individuals have an increased tendency to develop malignancy. These include a number of non-AIDS defining malignancies, as well as the AIDS defining malignancies which are Kaposi sarcoma, invasive cervical cancer and non-Hodgkin Lymphoma (NHL). Among the NHL group, the incidence of systemic NHL, CNS Lymphoma and primary effusion lymphoma are increased in this population. Malignancies continue to be an important cause of mortality in these individuals.

The incidence of NHL increases with progressive immunosuppression in HIV-infected patients. The majority of these cases are intermediate or high-grade and almost all are diffuse large B cell (immunoblastic variant) or Burkitt-like lymphomas. The incidence of Hodgkin lymphoma (HL) is also increased in the HIV positive population (Bigar R et al, 2006) though it is not an AIDS defining illness. Acute myeloid leukemia may also occur with higher frequency in the setting of HIV infection (Grulich A et al, 2007). NHL and HL occurring in HIV infected individuals are characterized by an aggressive clinical course with an advanced stage at presentation (Levine AM, 2000).

In the pre-HAART era, the standard treatment for AIDS associated NHL was low dose chemotherapy. It was thought that they would be unable to tolerate intensive chemotherapy because of the underlying immunodeficiency. Randomized trials of standard doses of combination chemotherapy versus reduced doses revealed inferior results in the standard dose arm due to increased hematologic toxicity and infections (Kaplan LD et al, 1997). In the post-HAART era, patients were treated more aggressively due to improved hematologic reserve in patients on HAART. Patients are now treated similar to non HIV NHL patients.

Their remission rates and median survival with aggressive combination chemotherapy and HAART is similar to their HIV negative counterparts (Boue, F et al, 2006).

Consequently, more aggressive therapies such as high dose chemotherapy and stem cell transplantation have been explored in the HAART era with encouraging results. This chapter will go through autologous and allogeneic stem cell transplantation in HIV infected individuals and also highlight some of the recent developments in the field.

2. Autologous Stem Cell Transplantation (ASCT)

Autologous stem cell transplantation means transplantation with a person's own hematopoietic stem cells which are harvested ahead of time and cryopreserved for later use. Pluripotent hematopoietic stem cells are those which are capable of self renewal and of differentiation. These are the cells targeted for collection. The main advantage of this procedure is to enable the patient to receive myeloablative dose intense chemotherapy for a malignancy that has demonstrated a dose response to chemotherapy. Stem cells collected from the peripheral blood after priming with G-CSF (Granulocyte Colony Stimulating Factor) are generally preferred to stem cells from the bone marrow due to shorter engraftment times, thereby reducing morbidity and mortality. Stem cell apheresis is an outpatient procedure where cells are collected through large volume apheresis over approximately 4-6 hours. These stem cells are either cryopreserved with DMSO directly or can be manipulated by methods such as CD34 positive selection and transduction prior to cryopreservation.

There are various preparative regimens used for stem cell transplantation in patients with hematologic malignancy. The ideal regimen should be able to eradicate the malignancy, have no mortality and manageable side effects or toxicity. Alas, no such treatments exist. There are several treatment regimens in use. Selection of high dose chemotherapy regimens is based upon the use of chemotherapeutic agents that have a dose response in the hematologic malignancy. In addition, drugs are chosen that have nonoverlapping toxicities save for the hematologic toxicity. For example in NHL, typical agents include Cyclophosphamide, Etoposide, Carmustine (BCNU) and melphalan. In Hodgkin lymphoma, frequently utilized preparative regimens include the CBV regimen with Cyclophosphamide, Carmustine (BCNU), and Etoposide (VP-16) and the BEAM regimen with Carmustine (BCNU), Etoposide (VP-16), Cytarabine (Ara-C) and Melphalan.

Patients typically receive the conditioning regimen followed by infusion of thawed autologous stem cells approximately 24- 48 hours post completion of chemotherapy. Thereafter ensues a period of profound neutropenia, also often mucositis and GI toxicity such as nausea and diarrhea. During this period of neutropenia, the risk of infection is significantly increased. Hence patients are housed in hepa filtered rooms, and placed on low bacteria diets in addition to other infectious precautions. Nonetheless, fever and infection can be common. Mucositis is a risk factor for infection as it increases the likelihood of intermittent bacteremia from the GI tract. The use of peripheral blood progenitor cells harvested from apheresis instead of bone marrow stem cells led to a shortening of engraftment of white blood cell times.

This thereby reduced the period of neutropenia and mucositis, which improved survival in patients.

This procedure has been the standard treatment for HIV negative patients with relapsed NHL since the landmark PARMA trial published by Philip et al in the New England Journal of Medicine (1995). In this trial, patients with relapsed chemosensitive aggressive NHL were treated with 2 cycles of DHAP (Dexamethasone, Cisplatin and Cytarabine) and if responsive, randomly assigned to receive either DHAP for 4 additional cycles or high dose chemotherapy with BEAC (BCNU/Carmustine, Etoposide, Cytarabine and Cyclophosphamide) followed by ASCT, The results of this study revealed an overall survival (OS) benefit of 53 versus 32 percent (p= 0.038) in favor of the high dose chemotherapy arm. This approach has also been used in high risk patients who are in first remission (Haioun, C et al, 1997). Non-randomized trials of this high risk group have demonstrated high rates of progression free survival (FPS). Similarly, trials of HIV negative patients with Hodgkin Lymphoma have shown that ASCT can provide long term PFS for patients with relapsed disease (Linch, 1993). All these studies were done in the HIV negative population.

2.1. ASCT in HIV positive patients

ASCT in HIV positive patients was pioneered by the French in the pre-HAART era (Gabarre, J et al, 1996). The first patient was reported as a case study. He was a 40 year old male with HIV related NHL, receiving Zidovudine and Zalcitabine as antiretroviral treatment. He was treated with BEAM (BCNU, Etoposide, Cytarabine and Melphalan) chemotherapy for relapsed lymphoma followed by ASCT. His post-transplant course was complicated by several opportunistic infections including cytomegalovirus viremia, mycobacterium pneumonia and cryptosporidiosis. This report corroborated the fear that the immune impairment due to HIV augmented the infection risk. However, it also demonstrated that mobilizing stem cells and successful engraftment were feasible in this setting. In the post-HAART era, French investigators performed a study with fourteen patients with relapsed or refractory NHL. Eight patients died of which six deaths were from lymphoma. This study established that the mortality due to infection was substantially reduced, but that control of the underlying lymphoma remained the challenge (Gabarre et al, 2001). It set the stage for ASCT to be considered a feasible task in HIV patients, and revealed that infectious issues were manageable without apparent adverse consequences on the HIV infection.

Other centers have described similar findings. The larger City of Hope study had patients with less advanced lymphoma and disqualified chemotherapy refractory patients (Krishnan A, et al, 2005). The initial series consisted of 20 patients with HL or NHL. All patients were on HAART. The majority of patients underwent CBV (cyclophosphamide, BCNU, Etoposide) chemotherapy as conditioning. Engraftment times were comparable to HIV negative patients, median was 11 days. Despite efforts to continue HAART throughout the transplant period, only nine out of twenty were able to tolerate it. The remainder resumed it at a median of two months following ASCT. The poor tolerance of HAART was due to either nausea or mucositis. Transplant related mortality was low, as was the incidence of opportunistic infections. No patient died of an opportunistic infection. Although the CD4 count did nadir at 6 months, post-transplant follow up demonstrated that the underlying HIV disease did not deteriorate as a result of the transplant and the CD4 counts recovered to pre-transplant levels by one year in all patients. PFS and OS were 85%. The improved result compared to the French experience may be from selecting patients with less advanced disease and chemotherapy sensitive disease.

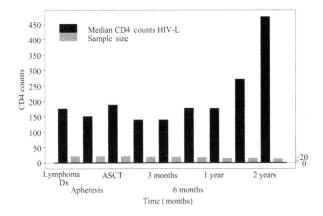

Figure 1. Median CD4 count trends during apheresis and after ASCT. Krishnan A et al. Blood 2005; 105:874-878 Blood: Journal of the American Society of Hematology by American Society of Hematology. Copyright 2009 Reproduced with permission of AMERICAN SOCIETY OF HEMATOLOGY (ASH) in the format Journal via Copyright Clearance Center.

The Italian cooperative group on AIDS and tumors (GIGAT) reported the long term results on 50 patients with HIV and relapsed or refractory lymphoma (Re A, et al, 2009). Similar to the City of Hope study, only patients with chemotherapy sensitive disease were selected to proceed with peripheral stem cell collection. Forty-six patients were already on HAART, two started at the time of study enrollment, and two at the time of stem cell mobilization. A minimum CD4 count of 100 cells/micro liter prior to initiating chemotherapy was a prerequisite. There were no eligibility criteria for viral load and therefore the viral loads at study entry ranged considerably. Thirteen patients withdrew before stem cell collection. Among these, two withdrawals were from early toxic deaths, one patient refusal, and the remaining ten patients had chemotherapy refractory disease. Eventually, twenty seven patients underwent ASCT. Of these, seven temporarily suspended HAART, some for similar reasons to the City of Hope experience with mucositis, and others for hepatotoxicity. All patients received BEAM (Carmustine/BCNU, Etoposide, Cytarabine and Melphalan) as the conditioning regimen. Three year progression free survival for the patients who proceeded to transplant was also similar to the City of Hope experience at 76.3%. Multivariate analysis of prognostic factors for survival showed that bone marrow involvement, performance status less than 2, and CD4 count below 100 cells/micro liter were significant. No significant HIV-associated infections were noted. In those patients on effective HAART therapy, the infectious risk was similar to patients without HIV who underwent ASCT. The high patient withdrawal rate before transplantation displays the obstacles in treating these aggressive lymphomas.

The European Group for Blood and Marrow Transplantation conducted a retrospective, multicentre registry-based analysis of sixty eight patients from twenty institutions since 1999 (Balsalobre P et al, 2009). There were fifty patients with NHL and eighteen patients with HL. At the time of ASCT, sixteen patients were in first complete remission (CR1); forty four patients were in CR more than 1, partial remission, or chemotherapy-sensitive relapse; and eight patients had chemotherapy resistant disease. Most patients were treated with a chemotherapy based conditioning regimen (BEAM and variants). The median CD4 count at transplantation was 162 cells/micro litter, and eighty percent of patients had an HIV viral load under 200/mL. All patients engrafted at a median of eleven days, save one. The incidence of non relapse mortality (NRM) was 4.4% and 7.5% at 3 and 12 months, respectively. Three patients died from bacterial infection, two died of HIV related complications, and one patient died of an unknown cause while in CR. At a median follow-up of 32 months, progression free survival and overall survival were 56.5% and 61% at three years, respectively. On multivariate analysis, chemotherapy resistant disease and not attaining complete remission predicted poorer progression free survival and overall survival. This data indicates again similar to the HIV negative transplant setting, disease control with chemotherapy at the time of ASCT predicts a more favorable result.

Two case control studies also demonstrated that HIV status does not impact ASCT outcomes for lymphoma. The European Group for Blood and Marrow Transplantation undertook a retrospective study of 106 patients (Diez-Martin et al, 2009) which included 53 HIV-positive lymphoma patients who underwent transplant with controls matched for histology, non-age adjusted IPI (International Prognostic Index), and disease status at transplant. There were 66 percent NHL and 34 percent HL patients. Both groups were similar, other than the higher percentage of males, mixed cellularity Hodgkin lymphoma and patients receiving granulocyte colony stimulating factor before engraftment, and a smaller fraction receiving total body irradiation based conditioning within the HIV lymphoma cohort. With median follow-up of 30 months, progression free survival was 61 percent for the HIV-lymphoma group and 56 percent for the control lymphoma group. Overall survival was 61.5 percent for HIV-positive patients and 70 percent for controls (p = NS). There was a trend towards delay in platelet engraftment after transplant in the HIV group. It is uncertain whether this resulted from the more frequent granulocyte colony stimulating factor use in that cohort or to HAART therapy or to chronic HIV infection of the bone marrow. Incidence of relapse, overall survival and progression free survival were comparable in both groups. In the first year following ASCT, there was an elevated, but statistically insignificant non relapse mortality in the HIV lymphoma group, primarily from early bacterial infections. This data suggested that in the HAART era, HIV infection should not preclude lymphoma patients from undergoing ASCT. The authors recommended conscientious infection prophylaxis and vigilant immune recovery surveillance shortly following ASCT.

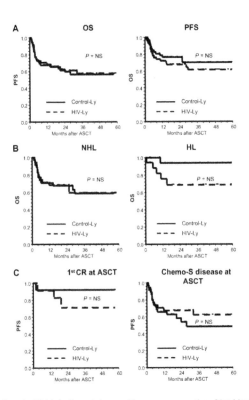

Figure 2. Survival according to HIV infection status: positive versus negative. Diez-Martin JL et al. Blood 2009; 113:6011-6014 Blood: Journal of the American Society of Hematology by American Society of Hematology. Copyright 2009 Reproduced with permission of AMERICAN SOCIETY OF HEMATOLOGY (ASH) in the format Journal via Copyright Clearance Center

City of Hope undertook a retrospective matched case-control study (Krishnan, et al, 2010) to study long-term outcome in HIV positive NHL patients (cases) and HIV negative NHL patients (controls). Twenty nine patients with HIV positive NHL were matched with HIV negative NHL controls with respect to sex, time to ASCT, year of transplant, histology, age, disease status, number of prior regimens, and conditioning regimen. A higher ratio of HIV positive NHL patients had high grade disease versus the HIV negative NHL controls. There were mostly male patients in both groups. The median CD4 count at study entry was 153.5, and the viral load was 6500. All patients in the HIV cohort were on HAART at the time of transplant; however thirteen patients had to interrupt treatment. The median follow-up for HIV-positive NHL patients was 62.4 months, and 48.4 months for the HIV-negative NHL controls. The median time to neutrophil engraftment was comparable for both groups. Non relapse mortality was also comparable for the two groups. Infectious complications did differ between the two groups, with more opportunistic infections occurring in the HIV-positive cohort, however this did not affect survival. There were more opportunistic viral infections in the HIV-positive group, with three cases of cytomegalovirus viremia, one case of adenovirus viremia, and one case of varicella infection. Disease free survival and overall survival were not significantly different between the two groups. The two year disease free survival for the HIV-positive NHL group was 76 percent and 56 percent for the HIV-negative group. The overall survival for both groups was also similar at 75 percent notwithstanding a higher proportion of poor risk HIV positive NHL patients.

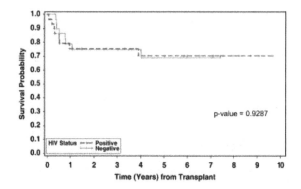

Figure 3. Probability of overall survival by HIV status. Krishnan A, Palmer J, Zaia J, et al. Vol. 16, (September 2010), pp. 1302-08. "Reprinted From: HIV Status Does Not Affect the Outcome of Autologous Stem Cell Transplantation (ASCT) for Non-Hodgkin Lymphoma (NHL) Biology of Blood and Marrow Transplantation 16:1302-1308 (2010), with permission from Elsevier"

Causes of death in the HIV-positive cohort were mostly from relapsed lymphoma, and not infection. Disease status at the time of transplant was the only clear predictor of outcome. This single-institution series corroborates the European data.

This data from the European Group for Blood and Marrow Transplantation (Balsalobre et al, 2009) and the City of Hope experience (Krishnan, et al, 2010) revealed better progression free survival rates in the HIV-positive lymphoma patients compared to their HIV-negative counterparts. This improved early outcome is interesting. Perhaps incorporating HAART in the regimen improves the result. Maybe transplant with high dose chemotherapy resets the clock on the immunologic effects of HIV, either by depleting the HIV reservoir or by its alterations on the T cell reconstitution. Inherent genetic variability may also play a part. Homozygosity for the 32-bp CCR5 allele CCR-Δ 32 has been shown to confer resistance to HIV infection (Liu R et al, 1996). This same deletion may also offer defense against lymphoma development in HIV patients (Dean M et al, 1999). A trial in the United States of ASCT for HIV lymphoma via the Bone Marrow Transplant Clinical Trials Network will prospectively analyze the genotypes and the CCR5 mutation to find its association with disease free survival. Correlative studies will also assess the pre and post-transplant HIV viral reservoir.

2.2. Immune recovery post transplant

An Italian study (Simonelli et al, 2010) prospectively evaluated 33 lymphoma patients of whom 24 were HIV positive and nine were HIV-negative. All patients had relapsed or refractory disease and both groups were given similar high dose chemotherapy and ASCT protocols. The study compared the immunological baseline features in the two groups. The study showed that front line chemotherapy resulted in immunodepression in the general population, which qualitatively differs from that observed in HIV-infected patients. HIV-positive patients had higher CD8+ T cell counts and inverted ratios of CD4+ cells to CD8+ cells than HIV-negative patients. There were no significant differences in the CD4+ cell compartment and thymic reservoir, between the groups. The authors attributed this finding to good control of HIV-RNA levels from ongoing HAART therapy. The initial differences in the dynamics of immune recovery between the populations also diminished with longer follow-up. Specifically, the CD8+ subpopulation, together with CD56+ NK cells quickly recovered in both groups of patients, leading, to a reversal of the ratio of CD4+ cells to CD8+ cells in the HIV-negative patients for up to two years following transplantation. In the HIV-infected population, high dose chemotherapy produced a different immune incompetence compared with conventional chemotherapy, which primarily impacted the CD4+ T cell subset without significantly affecting the CD4/CD8 ratio. In the first three months post ASCT, significantly more infectious episodes occurred in the HIV-positive group. The authors demonstrated that HIV-positive patients with early post-transplant infections had significantly lower CD4+ T cell counts during the third month post ASCT, compared with HIV-negative patients without infections. There was no difference in the frequency of infection or the dynamics of CD4+ T cell reconstitution beyond three months post ASCT. Overall, the study showed that high dose chemotherapy and ASCT in HIV-infected lymphoma patients does not worsen initial immune impairment or enhance viral replication or peripheral HIV reservoir in the long term. The temporary elevation in the incidence of early infectious events in the HIV-positive group may be related to an arrest in the CD4+ T cell count increment during the first three months post ASCT. There were no significant changes in the HIV DNA levels during the follow-up period, with values at 24 months significantly lower than those at baseline.

It is well-recognized that HIV persists at low levels in peripheral blood mononuclear cells, mostly in infected resting CD4+ T cells which constitute a stable reservoir for HIV, even when viral replication is well controlled with antiretroviral therapy. Analysis of HIV-1 DNA (HIV DNA) (Koelsch, KK et al, 2008) in peripheral blood mononuclear cells is therefore an accessible virological marker for estimating HIV infection. Bortolin's study of 22 patients with HIV associated relapsed or refractory lymphomas treated with salvage high dose chemotherapy followed by ASCT looked at the kinetics of the predictive value of HIV DNA. HIV DNA was measured by real-time PCR in the peripheral blood mononuclear cells. At baseline, HIV DNA was found to be associated with HIV-1 RNA (HIV RNA), but not with CD4 counts. HIV RNA load was under control throughout follow-up, while HIV DNA levels were nearly always detectable. The overall survival analysis demonstrated that patients with higher HIV DNA levels at baseline had a higher and nearly significant risk of death when compared with patients with lower levels (HR, 8.33, 95% CI 0.99 - 70.06, p=0.05). At the time of publication, of the 22 patients, 14 (63.6%) were still alive, of which 13 were in remission and one relapsed; 8 (36.5%) died, of which 6 deaths were from relapsed lymphoma and 2 were from opportunistic infections. Of note, baseline HIV DNA levels were significantly different between alive and deceased patients. Results from this study established HIV DNA as an valuable additional tool to optimize and tailor therapy, and also predict treatment outcome in these patients.

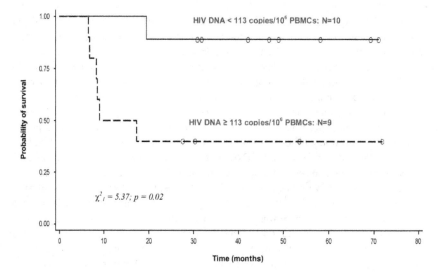

Figure 4. Kaplan–Meier curve showing survival according to baseline HIV DNA levels (*n* = 19) Bortolin MT, Zanussi S, Talamini R, et al. *AIDS Research and Human Retroviruses*. Vol. 26, No. 2, (2010), pp. 245-251. " The publisher for this copyrighted material is Mary Ann Liebert, Inc. publishers."

3. Allogeneic transplantation

Allogeneic transplantation refers to hematopoietic stem cells which come from an HLA matched donor. Allogeneic transplants typically have a higher morbidity and mortality than autologous transplants mostly due to infection or graft versus host disease. The 'graft' refers to the transplanted hematopoietic stem cells transplanted from the donor (sibling or matched unrelated donor) and the 'host' refers to the patient. In graft versus host disease, the donor's immune cells attack the recipient's organs. Virtually any organ can be affected, but frequently affected organs include the skin, liver and gut. Graft versus host disease (GVHD) is a major impediment to the success of bone marrow transplantation. Treatment and prevention of GVHD includes immunosuppressive medications and sometimes steroids. The incidence of chronic graft versus host disease (that occurring after 100 days post transplant) is up to 80% in recipients of allogeneic peripheral blood stem cells. On the other hand, allogeneic transplant has the advantage of lower rates of relapse due to the 'clean graft' as well as the immunologic effects of the donor graft, the so called graft versus tumor effect. These immunologic effects could be potentially even more beneficial in the treatment of HIV infection if the attendant risks of the procedure in the HIV infected patient could be overcome.

Allogeneic stem cell transplantation (alloSCT) is more difficult than ASCT in HIV infected individuals due to the need for chronic immunosuppression in an already immunosuppressed individual. Solid organ transplantation set the stage for allogeneic stem cell transplantation in that solid organ transplant patients also need chronic immunosuppression. There have been several published reports of solid-organ transplantation in HIV positive patients who are receiving HAART, which demonstrated that, in most cases, HIV infection does not affect the outcome of transplantation. Drug interactions were handled by requisite dose adjustments. The underlying HIV infection was controlled provided patients remained on antiretroviral therapy. (Ragni MV et al, 1999; Prachalias AA et al, 2001; Kuo PC, 2001; Gow PJ & Mutimer D, 2001 as cited in Halpern et al, 2002). Some solid organ transplant centers regard HIV patients akin to other high risk patients, for example, diabetics, or the elderly (Persad G et al, 2008).

The literature on allogeneic transplantation in HIV positive patients is considerably more limited than ASCT. Experience with ASCT in HIV-positive patients has shown that HIV infection did not impede engraftment provided myelosuppressive medications like azidothymidine were avoided. Therefore, in the allogeneic field, comparable engraftment times were expected. Allogeneic transplantation data indicates the rate of immune reconstitution after transplant is related to the type of conditioning regimen, HLA compatibility of the donor and host, and the occurrence of GVHD. In an allogeneic transplant with an HIV negative recipient, T lymphocyte recovery occurs by thirty days following transplant, although initially with primarily CD8+ T cells (Keever, CA et al, 1989). CD4+ cell recovery often takes up to six months.

Early reports of allogeneic transplant were in the pre-HAART period. Holland et al (1989) at Johns Hopkins published a case of a forty one year old male with HIV lymphoma who received a conditioning regimen consisting of total body irradiation and Cyclophosphamide followed by allogeneic bone marrow transplantation. Prior to the transplant, he was given high dose azidothymidine and following the transplant, he was given a lower dose. There was no significant regimen-related toxicity, and he engrafted at day seventeen, but thereafter died of lymphoma at day forty seven. At autopsy, no evidence of HIV, either by culture, or PCR was found in tissue specimens. Although the result was poor, this early report demonstrated the achievability of the procedure and raised the intriguing question, could allogeneic transplant be a route to treat HIV infection.

Woolfrey et al (2008) published a series of two HIV-positive patients who received nonmyeloablative transplants at the Fred Hutchinson Research Center. They received conditioning with Fludarabine and 200 cGy total body irradiation. They got HLA-matched peripheral blood stem cells, one from a sibling and the other from an unrelated donor. Post-transplantation cyclosporine and mycophenolatemofetil were given for graft versus host disease prophylaxis. HAART was continued with adjustments to prevent drug interactions. The HIV RNA remained undetectable and no HIV associated infections were noted. The first patient died of GVHD. The second patient remained alive at the time of publication, more than 180 days following transplant. It is notable that both patients' donor cells expressed wild-type CCR5 co receptor, and not the CCRΔ32 allele which is linked with resistance to HIV infection. Reconstitution of CD4+ and CD8+ subsets was in accordance with other nonmyeloablative transplants. New HIV-1 specific CD8+ T cell responses were produced after transplant. The gradual loss of detectable proviral DNA in the patient who achieved full donor chimerism suggests that the reservoir of latently infected lymphocytes died out after transplantation. This study alluded to the dual benefits of allogeneic transplantation.

Larger studies are needed to determine if the benefits of allogeneic transplant can be preserved in the myeloablative setting with its accompanying elevated morbidity and mortality. The largest series was a retrospective study of thirty patients with various hematologic malignancies transplanted between 1987 and 2003 from the European Group for Blood and Marrow Transplantation (Gupta V, et al, 2007). Treatment related mortality at 100 days was 46 percent. There was a striking difference in survival in patients transplanted after 1996 after availability of HAART. Prior to 1996, only two out of twenty two patients survived, but after 1996, four out of eight patients survived. This study revealed that reduction of transplant related mortality and control of HIV infection together are imperative in carrying out successful allogeneic transplants in this population.

4. Allogeneic transplantation for HIV infection

Allogeneic hematopoietic stem cell transplantation has the exciting prospect of controlling the HIV infection. HIV-1 enters host cells by binding to a CD4 receptor and then interacting with either CCR5 or the CXC chemokine receptor (CXCR4). Homozygosity for a 32-bp deletion (delta 32) in the CCR5 allele confers natural resistance to infection with CCR5 tropic HIV strains (R5 HIV) because of the lack of CCR5 cell-surface expression. (Dean M et al, 1996 as cited in Allers et al, 2011)

A case report from Germany by Hutter et al (2009) published in the *New England Journal of Medicine* described a 40 year old patient with a ten year history of HIV who underwent allogeneic stem cell transplantation (SCT) in February 2007 for relapsed acute myelogenous leukemia from an HLA-matched unrelated donor who was homozygous for the CCR5 delta 32 allele. HAART was given until the day prior to transplantation. The patient relapsed at day 332 and was treated with a second transplant from the same donor after reinduction therapy with cytarabine and gemtuzumab along with single dose total body irradiation. There was no viral rebound twenty months after transplantation and discontinuation of antiretroviral therapy. Tissue sites, such as the intestines, serve as reservoirs, and were looked at to detect the HIV virus despite the absence of viremia. In this patient, the rectal biopsy performed at 159 days after transplant did reveal that CCR5-producing macrophages were still present in the intestinal mucosa, which demonstrated they had not yet been replaced by the new immune system. Although these long-lasting cells from the host can be viral reservoirs even after transplantation, HIV-1 DNA was not found in his rectal mucosa. Immunologic studies showed a loss of anti-HIV virus specific interferon gamma producing T cells. This indicated that HIV antigenic stimulation was not present post transplant. His viral load continued to be undetectable despite the presence of non-CCR5 tropic X4 virus variants. After nearly two years of follow-up, the patient's CD4 cell count normalized with all cells exhibiting the homozygous CCR5-deleted gene. This observation is notable because homozygosity for CCR5 delta 32 deletion is related to high but not complete resistance to HIV-1.

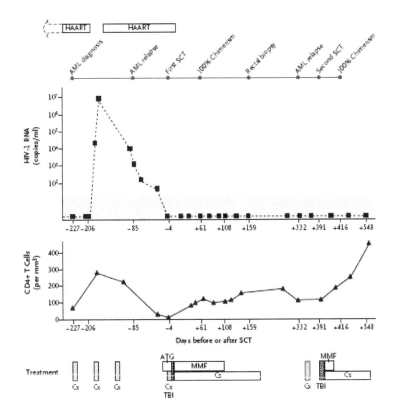

Figure 5. Clinical Course and HIV-1 Viremia. Hütter G, Nowak D, Mossner M, et al. Long-term control of HIV by CCR5 Delta32/Delta32 stem-cell transplantation. *The New England Journal of Medicine,* Vol. 360, No. 7, (February 2009) pp. 692-8. Permission granted. Copyright MMS

Allers et al (2011) published an article involving the same patient with extended follow-up, which reveals that he had remained off HAART and had no evidence of HIV disease for 45 months after the transplant. During his treatment course, he underwent multiple colonoscopies with biopsies to rule out GVHD, in addition to a liver biopsy and brain biopsy for evaluation of leukoencephalopathy. This study also looked at 10 HIV negative stem cell transplant controls and 15 HIV negative healthy controls, 5 of whom underwent colonoscopy as a cancer preventive examination. It was found that CD4+ T cell reconstitution increased continuously and, after two years reached levels within the normal range of age matched healthy patients. There was 100 percent donor chimerism, which was shown by absent CCR5 expression. Among the CD4+ T cells, there were more activated effector memory cells and less naïve cells when compared with healthy controls. CD4+ T cell reconstitution also occurred in the gut mucosa of the reported patient, similar to the stem cell transplant control patients, with cells exclusively derived from the donor hematopoietic system. There was more than a twofold increase in mucosal CD4+ T cells in the transplant patients compared to healthy controls, which demonstrates that conditioning and transplant elicits the enrichment of HIV target cells in the gut mucosal immune system.

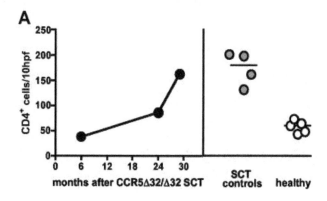

Figure 6. The mucosal immune system has been efficiently repopulated with donor-derived CD4+ T cells. (A) Immuno-histochemical quantification of CD4+ T cells in colon tissue of the CR5Δ32/Δ32 SCT patient, SCT control patients (27 ± 9 months after transplantation), and healthy control patients. The horizontal lines denote the median values of each group. Allers K, Hütter G, Hofmann J, et al. *Blood.* Vol. 117, No. 10, (March 2011), pp. 2790-2799. Blood: journal of the American Society of Hematology by American Society of Hematology. Copyright 2009 Reproduced with permission of AMERICAN SOCIETY OF HEMATOLOGY (ASH) in the format Journal via Copyright Clearance Center

HIV RNA and DNA were not detected in the peripheral blood or biopsy specimens obtained from various tissues. These biopsies revealed that tissue macrophages were ultimately replaced by donor-derived macrophages without CCR5 expression (Parker and Sereti, 2011). The T cells of the reported patient do not express normal levels of CXCR4 and appear vulnerable to X4-tropic HIV. HIV specific antibodies declined over time, with only envelope antibodies being detectable at the time of publication.

The study suggests that CCR5Δ32/Δ32 SCT has probably led to a cure of HIV infection in this patient. However it remains difficult to conclusively demonstrate eradication of HIV and its latent reservoirs, and the chance of resurgence of lingering X4 strains which survived the chemotherapy and radiation, leading to X4 HIV rebound still exists. Host-originating

CD4+ T cells appear to be totally removed from the immune system; however tissue macrophages are practically resistant to conditioning and less susceptible to the cytopathic effects of HIV infection, making them resilient viral reservoirs (Swingler S et al, 2007). One of the most promising findings of this report was the demonstration that later in the course of immune reconstitution, host-originating macrophages became undetectable in the GI mucosa by both phenotypic and genotypic analysis. These findings suggest that the replacement of host tissue cells with donor derived cells has reduced the size of the viral reservoir during the course of the immune reconstitution, which consequently had reduced the risk of HIV rebound over time.

5. Gene therapy and the future

Gooley et al (2010) reported impressive decreases in allogeneic transplantation-related mortality. Nevertheless, the risk of allogeneic SCT is inappropriately high to recommend it in the absence of an underlying malignancy that requires it as therapy. It cannot be proposed as a treatment strategy for the bulk of HIV-infected patients who can live long healthy lives with the use of HAART. Homozygosity for the delta 32 mutation is only found in a minority of the population, so it is not feasible to find such HLA-matched donors for the majority of patients. Preferably, one would aspire to integrate the benefits of transplantation of cells with the CCR5 mutation without the hazards of allogeneic SCT. One potential way to achieve this would be to transplant autologous stem cells that were genetically modified to be CCR5 negative. We have performed two trials at the City of Hope using this approach. The most recent employed a lentivirus-based system to transduce stem cells with a combination of three forms of anti-HIV RNA. This incorporated RNA1 in the form of a short-hairpin RNA targeted to an exon in HIV-1 tat/rev, a decoy for the HIV tat reactive element and a ribozyme that targets the host cell CCR5 chemokine receptor. Krishnan et al (2008) reported four patients with AIDS-related lymphoma transplanted with autologous lentiviral-transduced modified stem cells and unmanipulated stem cells following high-dose chemotherapy. All patients engrafted and exhibited low levels of genetically modified cells. Future trials will address how to augment engraftment of the genetically modified stem cells. Further plans are for planned interruption of HAART which would further demonstrate the functionality of these genetically modified cells. It is likely that an amalgamation of approaches with an aim to limit CD4 T cell targets and target viral reservoirs may be necessary to achieve a cure.

6. Conclusion

In the HAART era, the barrier of HIV infection as an obstacle to transplant has been broken. The role of ASCT has been well established in the HIV negative population for the treatment of relapsed or high-risk lymphoma. Numerous studies have now shown that ASCT can be safely performed in HIV-positive patients, and that it may lead to durable remissions in patients with HIV-related lymphomas. Similar to well controlled diabetes, well controlled HIV infection does not significantly increase the risk of infections following ASCT if a program of adequate surveillance and prophylaxis is used. Allogeneic stem cell transplantation remains a more difficult task, is still in its infancy, and lacks larger studies. The Hutter and Allers experience of allogeneic SCT with a CCR5 negative donor has given a name and face to the cure of HIV. The task of finding more feasible options for the enormousglobal population living with HIV remains.

Author details

Nitya Nathwani

City of Hope National Medical Center, Duarte, USA

References

[1] Allers, K., Hütter, G., Hofmann, J., et al., & (2011, . (2011). Evidence for the cure of HIV infection by CCR5 (Delta) 32 (Delta) 32 stem cell transplantation.Blood. March 2011), , 117(10), 2790-2799.

[2] Balsalobre, P., Diez-Martin, J., Re, A., et al. (2009). Autologous stem-cell transplantation in patients with HIV-related lymphoma. Journal of Clinical OncologyMay 2009), , 27(13), 2192-2198.

[3] Biggar, R., Jaffe, E., Goedert, J., et al. (2006). Hodgkin Lymphoma and immunodeficiency in persons with HIV/AIDS. BloodDecember 2006, , 108(12), 3786-3791.

[4] Bortolin, M. T., Zanussi, S., Talamini, R., et al. (2010). Predictive value of HIV Type 1 DNA levels on overall survival in HIV-related lymphoma patients treated with high-dose chemotherapy (HDC) plus autologous stem cell transplantation (ASCT). *AIDS Research and Human Retroviruses*, 26(2), 245-251.

[5] Boue, F., Gabarre, J., Gisselbrecht, C., et al. (2006). Phase II trial of CHOP Plus Rituximab in Patients With HIV_Associated Non-Hodgkin's Lymphoma. Journal of Clinical Oncology.September 2006) , 24(25), 4123-4128.

[6] Dean, M., Jacobson, L. P., Mc Farlane, G., et al. (1999). Reduced risk of AIDS lymphoma in individuals heterozygous for the CCR5-DELTA32 mutation. Cancer Research-August 1999), , 3561-2564.

[7] Díez-Martín, J. L., Balsalobre, P., Re, A., et al. (2009). Comparable survival between HIV+ and HIV- non-Hodgkin and Hodgkin lymphoma patients undergoing autologous peripheral blood stem cell transplantation. *Blood*. 113. June 2009), (23), 6011-6014.

[8] Forman SJ, Blume KG, Thomas ED,(1994). Bone Marrow Transplantation.Blackwell Scientific Publications. 0-86542-253-2

[9] Gabarre, J., Choquet, S., Azar, N., et al. (2001). High Dose Chemotherapy with autologous stem cell transplantation for HIV associated lymphoma: A single center report on 14 patients. Blood 2001; 98: Abstract # 2092

[10] Gabarrre, J., Leblond, V., Sutton, L., et al. (1996). Autologous bone Marrow transplantation in relapsed HIV related Non-Hodgkin's lymphoma. Bone Marrow Transplantation 1996; 18: , 1195-1197.

[11] Gooley TA, Chien JW, Pergam SA, et al(2010). Reduced mortality after allogeneic hematopoietic-cell transplantation. The New England Journal of MedicineNovember 2010), , 363(22), 2091-2101.

[12] Grulich AE, Leeuwen MT, Falster MO, et al.(2007). Incidence of cancers in people with HIV/AIDS compared with immunosuppressed transplant recipients: a meta-analysis. Lancet. July 2007), , 370, 59-67.

[13] Gupta, V., Tomblyn, M., Pederson, T., et al. (2007). Allogeneic hematopoietic stem cell transplantation in HIV-positive patients with malignant and non-malignant disorders: a report from the center for international blood and marrow transplant research (CIBMTR). Biology of Blood and Marrow TransplantationSupplement, (February 2007) , 13(2), 5-6.

[14] Haioun, C., Lepage, E., Gisselbrecht, C., et al. (1997). Benefit of autologous bone marrow transplantation over sequential chemotherapy in poor risk aggressive non-Hodgkin's lymphoma: Updated results of the Prospective Study LNH87-2. Journal of Clinical OncologyMarch 1997), , 15(3), 1131-1137.

[15] Halpern SD, Ubel PA &Caplan AL(2002). Solid Organ Transplantation in HIV infected patients. The New England Journal of MedicineJuly 2002), , 347(4), 284-287.

[16] Holland, H. K., Saral, R., Rossi, J. J., et al. (1989). Allogeneic bone marrow transplantation, zidovudine and human immunodeficiency virus type 1 (HIV-1) infection. Annals of Internal Medicine.111(12) (December 1989), , 973-981.

[17] Hütter, G., Nowak, D., Mossner, M., et al. (2009). Long-term control of HIV by CCR5 Delta32/Delta32 stem-cell transplantation. The New England Journal of Medicine-February 2009) , 360(7), 692-698.

[18] Kaplan, LD, Strauss DJ, Testa, MA et al.(1997). Low-Dose Compared with Standard-Dose m-BACOD Chemotherapy for Non-Hodgkin's Lymphoma Associated with Human Immunodeficiency Virus Infection.The New England Journal of Medicine.June 1997) , 336, 1641-1648.

[19] Keever, Small. T. N., Flomenberg, N., et al. (1989). Immune Reconstitution following bone marrow transplantation: Comparison of recipients of T cell depleted marrow with recipients of conventional marrow grafts. BloodApril 1989) , 73(5), 1340-1350.

[20] Koelsch, K. K., Liu, L., Haubrich, R., et al. (2008). Dynamics of total, linear noninte-grated, and integrated HIV-1 DNA in vivo and in vitro. The Journal of Infectious Dis-eases. 197 (February 2008), , 411-419.

[21] Krishnan, A., Molina, A., Zaia, J., et al. (2005). Durable Remissions with autologous stem cell transplantation for high-risk HIV associated lymphomas. BloodJanuary 2005), , 105(2), 874-878.

[22] Krishnan, A., Palmer, J., Zaia, J., et al. (2010). HIV status does not affect the outcome of autologous stem cell transplantation (ASCT) for Non-Hodgkin Lymphoma (NHL). Biology of Blood and Marrow TransplantationSeptember 2010), , 16, 1302-1308.

[23] Krishnan, A., Zaia, J. A., Rossi, J., et al. (2008). First in Human Engraftment of Anti HIV lentiviral vector gene modified CD 34+ peripheral blood progenitor cells in the treatment of AIDS related lymphoma (ARL). Blood. 112: Abstract 2348

[24] Levine AM.(2000). Acquired immunodeficiency Syndrome-Related Lymphoma: Clin-ical Aspects. Seminars in OncologyAugust 2000), , 27(4), 442-453.

[25] Linch, D. C., Goldstone, A. H., Mc Millan, A., et al. (1993). Dose intensification with autologous bone marrow transplantation in relapsed and resistant Hodgkin's dis-ease: results of a BNLI randomized trial. The Lancet. April 1993), , 341(8852), 1051-1054.

[26] Liu, R., Paxton, W., Choe, S., et al. (1996). Homozygous defect in HIV-1 coreceptor accounts for resistance of some multiply-exposed individuals to HIV-1 infection. Cel-lAugust 1996), , 86, 367-377.

[27] Palella FJ, Delaney KM, Moorman AC, et al.(1998). Declining morbidity and mortali-ty among patients with advanced human immunodeficiency virus infection. The New England Journal of MedicineMarch,1998), , 338(13), 853-860.

[28] Parker, R. ., Sereti, I., & (2011, . (2011). The power of 1 in HIV therapeutics.Blood. March 2011), , 117(10), 2745-2746.

[29] Persad, G. C., Little, R. F., & Grady, C. (2008). Including persons with HIV infection in cancer clinical trials. Journal of Clinical Onoclogy, March 2008), , 26(7), 1027-1032.

[30] Philip, T., Guglielmi, C., Hagenbeek, A., et al. (1995). Autologous bone marrow trans-plantation as compared with salvage chemotherapy in relapses of chemotherapy-sensitive non-Hodgkin's lymphoma. The New England Journal of Medicine. December 1995), , 333(23), 1540-1545.

[31] Re, A., Michieli, M., Casari, S., et al. (2009). High-dose therapy and autologous pe-ripheral blood stem cell transplantation as salvage treatment for AIDS-related lym-phoma: long-term results of the Italian Cooperative Group on AIDS and Tumors (GICAT) study with analysis of prognostic factors. BloodAugust 2009), , 114(7), 1306-1313.

[32] Simonelli, C., Zanussi, S., Pratesi, C., et al. (2010). Immune recovery after autologous stem cell transplantation is not different for HIV-infected versus HIV-uninfected pa-

tients with relapsed or refractory lymphoma. Clinical Infectious DiseasesJune 2010) , 1672-1679.

[33] Swingler, S., Mann, A. M., Zhou, J., et al. (2007). Apoptotic killing of HIV-1 infected macrophages is subverted by the viral envelope glycoprotein. PLoS PathogensSeptember 2007), , 3(9), 1281-1290.

[34] Woolfrey, A. E., Malhotra, U., Harrington, Rd., et al. (2008). Generation of HIV-1 specific CD8+ cell responses following allogeneic hematopoietic cell transplantation. Blood, October 2008), , 112(8), 3484-3487.

HIV Screening

Chapter 4

Screening for HIV Infection in Pregnancy

Chi Dola, Maga Martinez, Olivia Chang and
Amanda Johnson

Additional information is available at the end of the chapter

1. Introduction

Approximately 100 to 200 infants annually in the United States are infected with HIV (CDC, 2007). Most were born to mothers who were unaware of their infected HIV status or who did not receive preventative services during their pregnancy to reduce transmission rates. Therefore, in 2006, the CDC updated its guidelines for screening of various populations for HIV, including pregnant women. Obstetricians and gynecologists are ideally suited to such screening of their patients during annual exams and prenatal visits.

1.1. Screening for HIV infection during prenatal care

Screening only patients who reported risk factors for the HIV infection will miss many infected women. Therefore, the current recommendation is for implementation of universal opt-out screening for HIV as early in pregnancy as possible (Branson et al., 2006). In this universal opt-out screening method, a patient is informed that HIV testing will be performed as a routine part of her prenatal care, unless she declines testing. She should be given written or oral information about HIV, including an explanation of the infection, the meaning of positive or negative test results, and measures that can be used to reduce perinatal transmission. She should also be given the opportunity to ask further questions. However, no informed consent is required. If a patient declines screening, this should be documented in the medical record, and screening should be offered at subsequent prenatal visits (Branson et al., 2006; ACOG, 2008). Retesting is recommended with each new pregnancy. Although these are the recommendations endorsed by the CDC and ACOG, healthcare providers must be aware of the laws regarding screening in their own states, which may differ from the above guidelines. Further information on state HIV testing laws can be obtained from state and local health departments.

Chou et al, estimated that the number needed to screen (NNS) in an area with 0.15% prevalence would be between 3,500 to 12,170 to prevent 1 case of perinatally-acquired HIV infection. In a high risk area with a prevalence of 5%, the NNS would be from 105 to 365 to prevent 1 case of perinatally-acquired infection (Chou et, 2005).

At this time, both conventional and rapid screening tests for HIV are available to the healthcare provider. Conventional testing consists of a screening test with an enzyme immunoassay (ELISA), followed by confirmatory testing of a positive result with Western blot or immunofluorescent antibody (IFA) testing. The sensitivity and specificity of this method of testing is greater than 99%. False positive results are rare even in the setting with low prevalence. Final results may not be available for several days to weeks. With rapid testing, a blood or saliva test for HIV antibodies is performed, and the results are often available within an hour. Confirmatory testing of a preliminary positive result is still required before a diagnosis of HIV can be made. A negative result with either the conventional or rapid screening test indicates a woman does not have HIV, and no further testing is needed, unless one suspects the patient was recently infected with HIV but has not produced an antibody response to the virus (ACOG, 2008; Rahangdale & Cohan, 2008). If the initial screening test is positive, but the confirmatory test is negative, the patient should be considered not infected, and no further testing is necessary.

1.2. Rescreening in the third trimester

Studies from several countries have demonstrated that pregnant women seem to be at increased risk for acquisition of HIV over their non-pregnant counterparts (Moodley et al., 2009; Gray et al., 2005; Sansom et al., 2003). Theories for this range from behavioral actions of the woman or her partner that put her at increased risk, to physiologic changes associated with pregnancy, including changes to the genital tract mucosa to changes in cellular immunity that may lead to increased susceptibility to HIV with pregnancy. Evidence has demonstrated that the rate of seroconversion during pregnancy may be as high as 2 to 3 percent in some areas (Moodley et al., 2009; Gray et al., 2005; Sansom et al., 2003). A study by Sansom, *et al* demonstrated that in a population with an HIV incidence of approximately 1 in 1000 person-years, the cost of repeat testing was offset by the savings in medical costs for prevention of an infected infant (Sansom et al., 2003). For the above reasons, repeat HIV testing is recommended in certain populations in the third trimester, preferably before 36 weeks gestation (Branson et al., 2006; ACOG, 2008). These populations include:

- Women living in areas with a high incidence of HIV/AIDs, including the 20 states with the highest incidence among women of child-bearing age

- Women who receive their healthcare in facilities where at least 1 in 1000 women screened for HIV are found to be infected

- Women who engage in high-risk behavior that puts them at risk for HIV acquisition (injection drug use, exchange of sex for drugs or money, diagnosis of another sexually transmitted infection in the past year, a sex partner who engages in injection drug use or high-risk behaviors or is infected with HIV, or women who have had a new or more than one sexual partner during their pregnancy)

• Women with signs or symptoms of acute HIV infection

1.3. Screening of women with undocumented HIV status

Studies indicate that between 40 and 85 percent of infants infected with HIV are born to mothers whose HIV infection status is unknown prior to delivery (ACOG, 2008). If a woman without documentation of HIV status presents to labor and delivery, opt-out rapid HIV testing should be performed at time of her initial presentation. A positive result should prompt immediate treatment with antiretroviral prophylaxis without awaiting the result of confirmatory testing. If subsequent confirmatory testing shows the woman to be HIV negative, treatment may be discontinued. Similarly, if a woman has an unknown HIV status in the postpartum period, her infant should be tested by rapid screening. Antiretroviral treatment should be initiated with a positive result, as the benefits of such treatment are maximized when started within 48 hours of delivery (ACOG, 2008; Rahangdale & Cohan, 2008). Again, treatment may be stopped if confirmatory testing is negative.

The above recommendation for prenatal screening for HIV infection is summarized in table 1.

Timing	Screening test	Confirmatory Test
Initial prenatal care visit	Enzyme immunoassay (ELISA)	Western blot or immunofluorescent antibody (IFA) testing
Third trimester of pregnancy	Repeat ELISA in women at **high risk** for acquisition of HIV infection	Western blot or IFA testing
At time of labor and delivery for women with undocumented HIV status	Rapid HIV antibody screening test.	Western blot or IFA testing

Table 1. CDC and ACOG recommendation for screening for HIV infection during pregnancy.

2. Evidences supporting the effectiveness of current interventions to decrease mother-to-child transmission of HIV infection

Research in HIV infection reported several key factors in the transmission of the virus from the mother to the infant. The risk factors for transmission can be divided into: virologic/immunologic, maternal health status/behavior, and obstetrical factors (McGowan et al, 2000). High maternal plasma HIV-1 viral load, low maternal CD4 T-lymphocyte count, multidrug-resistant HIV genotype will increase the transmission rate. Certain maternal behavior (illicit drug use, cigarette smoking, breast feeding) or maternal health status (increased baseline weight or malnutrition or vitamin A deficiency) can increase the rate of mother-to-child transmission. Some obstetrical factors (vaginal delivery, prolonged rupture of membrane, fetal scalp electrode placement, chorioamnionitis, perineal lacerations, prematurity) can increase the vertical transmission rate (McGowan et al, 2000).

Other reports on perinatal transmission of HIV infection suggested that approximately 70% of the infections transmitted to the infant during the labor and delivery process; only 30% of the cases occurred during the antepartum period (Kourtis et al, 2006). Current interventions to prevent perinatal transmission of HIV infection included: prophylaxis therapy with antiretroviral medication, scheduled cesarean delivery and avoidance of breast feeding. These interventions resulted in decreasing transmission rate to 2% (Cooper et al, 2002). We will examine the evidence supporting these interventions.

2.1. Prophylaxis with antiretroviral agents

The Pediatric AIDS Clinical Trials Group (PACTG) 076 conducted a randomized controlled study and in 1994 published its landmark results demonstrating a reduction in perinatal HIV transmission by two-third with the antiretroviral medication Zidovudine (ZDV). HIV-infected mothers in the study group received a three-part regimen of antiretroviral medication. They received ZDV during pregnancy, intravenous ZDV during labor, and their infant received ZDV orally for 6 weeks (Conner et al, 1994). This trial reported a decrease in transmission rate from 26% in the placebo group to 8% in those patients who received ZDV. Later in the year of 1994, FDA approved the use of ZDV for reducing perinatal HIV transmission and the U.S. Public Health Service Task Force (USPHSTF) and CDC published their recommendations for the administration of this regimen in an effort to reduce mother-to-child transmission of the HIV infection (CDC, 2006).

In the late 1990s, additional antiretroviral medications were developed and the combined use of three or more of these drugs was found to greatly inhibit viral replication and allow improvement of the immune system. The combination of these medications was known as highly active antiretroviral therapy (HAART). In 1998, USPHSTF and CDC issued recommendation regarding HAART: pregnant women should receive HAART if they required the treatment for their disease status and all HIV-infected pregnant women should be offered HAART. USPHSTF and CDC at that time acknowledged that the benefits and risks to the fetus are uncertain (CDC, 1998). Four large U.S. and European cohort studies all concluded that regimens with two or more antiretroviral drugs were more effective than the one-drug regimen for reducing vertical transmission of the HIV infection (Cooper et al, 2002, Arch Pediatr Adolesc Med 2002, Clin Infect Dis 2005, Mandelbrot et al, 2001).

For women diagnosed late in pregnancy and were not able to receive a full course of antiretroviral treatment, a short course of antenatal treatment, although less effective, also was proven to decrease perinatal transmission (Lallemant et al, 2000, Shaffer et al, 1999, Petra study 2002, Wiktor et al, 1999, Dabis et al, 1999, Chou et al, 2005). There was some reduction in the HIV infection transmission even when treatment was abbreviated to only antiretroviral regimen during labor (Moodley et al, 2003, Taha et al, 2003, Guay et al, 1999). However,

neonatal prophylaxis alone in a mother who did not receive antiretroviral prophylaxis therapy was less effective in preventing HIV infection (Taha et al, 2003).

2.2. Scheduled cesarean delivery

A meta-analysis of 15 prospective cohort studies by the International Perinatal HIV
Group (The International Perinatal HIV Group, 1999) included 8,533 mother-neonate
pairs. Vertical HIV transmission was reduced by 50% when the mode of delivery was
elective cesarean delivery. The effect of both antiretroviral therapy prophylaxis and cesarean delivery further reduced HIV transmission by 87 percent when compared with
other modes of delivery (either vaginal delivery or non-elective cesarean delivery) and
no antiretroviral therapy. However, in women who received HAART and achieved
low HIV viral load levels (defined as less than 1,000 copies/ mL), current data is insufficient to determine whether elective cesarean delivery would offer further risk reduction. ACOG concluded that scheduled cesarean delivery should be discussed and
recommended for HIV-infected women whose HIV-1 RNA viral load exceeds 1,000
copies/mL. Scheduled cesarean delivery was recommended as early as 38 weeks gestation to reduce the risk of labor or of prematurely ruptured membranes (ACOG, 1999).

2.3. Avoidance of breastfeeding

Breastfeeding was associated with an HIV transmission rate of 14% to 16% based on the results of two meta-analyses of observational studies (Dunn et al, 1992, John et al, 2001). A review of the literature did not reveal any randomized, controlled trials evaluating the HIV
transmission rate associated with breastfeeding in the United States. A large, prospective cohort study in Italy included 3,770 babies and concluded that HIV infection rates were significantly higher in babies who were breastfed after the authors adjusted for other factors,
including antiretroviral use (adjusted odds ratio, 10.20 [CI, 2.73 to 38.11]) (Arch Pediatr Adolesc Med., 2002, Chou et al, 2005).

In a study in Africa, women who breastfed and did not receive antiretroviral therapy had a
probability of transmitting the HIV infection of 36.7% (CI, 29.4% to 44.0%) at 24 months and
an infant mortality rate of 24.4% (CI, 18.2% to 30.7%). Those who formula fed their babies
had a transmission probability of 20.5% (CI, 14.0% to 27.0%) and an infant mortality rate of
20.0% (CI, 14.4% to 25.6%) (Nduati et al, 2000).

As a result, in many countries, including the United States where formula feeding is readily
available and inexpensive, breastfeeding is not recommended for infants of HIV-infected
women (WHO, 2000).

3. Potential harms/risks as the result of prenatal HIV screening

We will next explore the potential risks as the results of prenatal HIV screening and the potential harms of the recommended interventions to reduce perinatal transmission of HIV infection (Table 2).

	Maternal risks	Fetal risks
Prenatal screening		
Screened positive	Discrimination from their partner Social ostracization from family and friends Anxiety and depression Abandonment and abuse from family and friend	
Screened falsely positive	Anxiety Social discrimination Relationship problems Unnecessary antiretroviral prophylaxis during labor	Potential risk for elective termination of pregnancy
Interventions to decrease perinatal transmission		
ART prophylaxis	Hepatic toxicity and hypersensitivity reaction (with Nevirapine) Development of drug resistance Gestational diabetes (with combination therapy including protease inhibitors)	Risks of neural tube defects with Sustive (Efavirenz) with first trimester exposure. ? Potential risk of mitochondrial toxicity and disorder Inconsistent data regarding increasing risk for preterm birth and low-birth weight
Scheduled cesarean delivery at 38 weeks	Post-operative morbidities, including: postpartum fever, hemorrhage, endometritis, urinary tract infection.	A trend toward higher risk of respiratory distress syndrome among neonates born by cesarean section (when compared to those born via vaginal delivery)

Table 2. Potential harms / risks from prenatal screening and strategic interventions to decrease perinatal transmission of HIV infection:

According to Katz, prenatal screening for HIV in pregnancy aims to test a presumably healthy population to discover asymptomatic women who are actually infected with HIV infection. These pregnant women might not have or perceive that they have risk factors for the HIV infection. This is different than the usual situation when a woman acknowledges her risk for the infection and requests the screening test. Most women would agree to be screened as they believe that they are doing everything they can for the health for their baby but they might not realize the full implication of a positive HIV test result on their lives. In some instances, they do not perceive that they are at risk for the infection and thus could be quite unprepared to receive the positive diagnosis. This could result in adverse effect on their emotional health, their pregnancy, and the family. Thus health care provider should always be well prepared to provide the appropriate emotional support for a possibility of abnormal result (Katz, 2000).

Women tested positive for HIV infection can experience significant problems with discrimination from their partner, social ostracization from their family and members of the community (Provisional Committee on Pediatric AIDS, 1995, Samson et al, 1998). They were found to have higher anxiety and depression scores and many women fear abandonment or abuse, therefore, did not disclose their HIV status to their friend or families. (Lester, 1995) although no increased risk for intimate partner violence was noted according to one cohort study (Koenig et al, 2002, Chou et al, 2005)

Data on consequences of false-positive HIV infection diagnoses in pregnant women are mainly anecdotal as reported by Sheon et al. The potential risks from false-positive results included: elective termination of pregnancy, anxiety, social discrimination and relationship problems with their partner (Sheon et al, 1994, Chou et al, 2005).

False positive results from rapid HIV testing during labor result in 4 women receiving unnecessary antiretroviral prophylaxis out of 4,849 women tested (Bulterys et al, 2004).

4. Risks of Antiretroviral Therapy (ART) to fetus

4.1. Potential teratogenic effects of ART

Efforts continue to increase our knowledge of the potential teratogenic effects of the antiretroviral agents administered in pregnancy. The Antiretroviral Pregnancy Registry Steering Committee published their recent report of antiretroviral exposures during pregnancy from January 1989 through July 2007. They did not identify an increased risk of birth defects in those exposed to any of the antiretroviral therapy in the first trimester. The risk of birth defects among women exposed to antiretroviral therapy in first trimester was 2.8 per 100 live births, which is not different from the risk of birth defects in women exposed to these agents in the second or third trimester (2.6 per 100 live births), nor the CDC's reported background rate of birth defects of 2.72 per 100 live births (www.APRegistry.com, 2007, Bardeguez, 2009).

Four retrospective reports associated Sustiva (Efavirenz) with neural tube defects in infants born of mothers exposed to this medication in the first trimester (Bardeguez, 2009). There are discrepant results with regard to mitochondrial toxicity and disorders in children exposed in utero to antiretroviral therapy. Two deaths believed to be due to mitochondrial disorder were reported in children exposed in utero to nucleoside analogues (in specific, a combination of Zidovudine and Lamivudine regimen) (Blanche et al, 1999). However, European Collaborative report and systematic review of U.S. cohorts reports did not find evidence of clinical symptoms, or deaths due to mitochondrial dysfunction among HIV-negative infants exposed to antiretroviral agents in utero (Bardeguez, 2009).

Of infants exposed in utero to Zidovudine who were followed at 4 years to 6 years of life. The reports were reassuring. Normal growth, cognitive, and developmental function were noted in these infants at 4 years old. They did not sustain any tumors or deaths from cancer at 6 years old.

4.2. Association between ART and preterm birth and low-birth weight

Inconsistent results were noted among the reports studying the effects of combination antiretroviral therapy on two obsterics outcomes: preterm birth and low birth-weight. Lorenzi et al in 1998 first reported the association between combination antiretroviral therapy with preterm birth in a retrospective Swiss study of 30 women (Lorenzi et al, 1998). Subsequently, other European studies reported a similar association between combination antiretroviral therapy and preterm birth (The European Collaborative Study (ECS) andSwiss Mother + Child HIV Cohort Study (Mo-CHiV), 2000, Grosch-Woerner et al, 2008). However, this association was not found in U.S. studies until a recent study by Cotter et al. The authors prospectively collected the data from 1990 through 2002 on 999 women receiving antiretroviral regimen during pregnancy. They concluded that women who received combination therapy that included a protease inhibitor had an increased risk of preterm delivery (Cotter et al, 2006).

In a largest analysis to date, Tuomola et al did not find an increased rate of premature birth or low birth-weight infants among 2,123 HIV infected pregnant women from seven clinical studies who received combination ART and gave birth from 1990 through 1998.

5. Risks of ART to mothers

A large prospective study evaluating the rates of maternal toxicity, pregnancy complications, and peripartum morbidity among HIV-infected pregnant women receiving prenatal care and ART concluded that adverse events were rare. Gestational diabetes was noted to be highest among women who received combination therapy including protease inhibitors either before or during first trimester (Watts et al, 2004). Reports of potential risks of hepatic toxicity and hypersensitivity reaction were noted in pregnant women receiving the drug Nevirapine (Bardeguez, 2009).

Another valid concern is the potential development of drug resistance when ART was administered to the mother for a short period during pregnancy. Drug resistance was noted in 20 – 69% of women who received only intrapartum prophylaxis with single-dose nevirapine. This could decrease the choice of medications for these women should they later need treatment for their disease. Although, there are reports that this observed resistance dissolved over time. (Bardeguez, 2009). Limited exposure to zidovudine alone did not alter maternal disease progression, time until development of AIDS or death, or development of genotypic zidovudine resistance (Bardeguez et al, 2003).

6. Potential maternal risks from scheduled cesarean delivery

Cesarean deliveries could result in significant complications when compared to vaginal delivery even for HIV-negative women (Allen et al., 2003; Makoha et al., 2004). HIV-infected women with an immunodeficient state could potentially at risk for post-operative infectious morbidities. Most studies report that HIV-infected women are at higher risk for post-operative complications, mostly infectious, than the uninfected women (Coll et al., 2002; Grubert el al., 1999; Vimercati et al., 2000). The rate of complications is higher in those with severe immunodeficiency (Jamieson et al., 2007).

Read et al conducted a largest prospective observational study which included 1,186 HIV-infected women from The Women and Infants Transmission Study. The authors evaluated the postpartum morbidity among these infected women according to their mode of delivery. When compared to women who delivered vaginally, women who underwent scheduled cesarean delivery had an increased rate of postpartum fever (14.3%), hemorrhage (7.1%), endometritis (5.4%), urinary tract infection (5.4%), and any postpartum morbidity (26.7%) (Read et al, 2001).

7. Potential neonatal risks from scheduled cesarean delivery at 38 weeks gestation

In the absence of medical or obstetrical indications, ACOG recommends against scheduled cesarean delivery at less than 39 weeks of gestation, due to the increased risk of respiratory morbidity in the neonate born prior to this gestational age (ACOG, 2001). Neonatal morbidity is high even among those neonates born via cesarean delivery a few days younger than 39 weeks (Tita et al, 2011). However, both ACOG and U.S. Public Health Service recommend scheduled cesarean delivery at 38 weeks for HIV-infected women with viral load greater than 1,000 copies/ml (ACOG, 2001; Public Health Service Task Force, 2010). The scheduled cesarean delivery date is set at one week earlier than the usually required gestational age of 39 weeks to avoid onset of spontaneous labor and rupture of membranes which could increase perinatal transmission of HIV. Livingston et al and the IMPACT Protocol 1025 Study Group evaluated the risk of neonatal respiratory distress syndrome according to the mode of delivery and gestational age at delivery. They reported that the mode of delivery was not associated with respiratory distress syndrome. However, there was a trend toward a higher risk of respiratory distress syndrome among neonates delivered by either elective or non-elective cesarean section when compared to those delivered vaginally. Two out of 227 neonates born via scheduled cesarean delivery at 38 weeks gestation had respiratory distress syndrome (Livingston et al., 2010).

8. Conclusion

Current evidence supports prenatal HIV screening. The benefits from screening appear to outweight the small risks / harms to the fetus and mothers from the treatment interventions which significantly reduce perinatal-acquired HIV infection. We concluded the chapter by discussing the obstacles to the HIV prenatal screening and prevention interventions. Prenatal screening for HIV infection and implementation of Protocol 076 were lauded as a major public health success story and resulted in a significant decline in the number of children infected with HIV from their mother. However, in the United States, there are still about 100–200 infants born every year with perinatally acquired HIV infection (CDC, 2007). Lack of prenatal care remains one of the obstacles to prevention of perinatal transmission of HIV. In the United States about 5 to 10% of women do not pursue prenatal care or receive insufficient care (Kogan et al., 1998). HIV infected women, in particular, often do not receive prenatal care. In New York City, 50% of women infected with HIV who delivered in at a municipal hospital did not receive prenatal care (Minkoff et al., 1990). Of the HIV-infected women surveyed in Philadelphia, only one third reported adequate prenatal care, and 20% did not receive any care (Turner et al., 1996).

Even more worrisome, at the Medical Center of Louisiana in New Orleans, LA, 50% of the HIV-infected parturients who did not have prenatal care but presented to the hospital for labor and delivery did not disclose their HIV status to their physicians (CDC, 2004). Could it be because the HIV-infected women did not know of the available interventions that they put their infants at risk for the infection?

Several authors attempt to understand why HIV-infected women opted out of prenatal care and available interventions to decrease vertical transmission. Rothpletz-Puglia et al solicited opinions from a group of HIV-negative women about the process of prenatal HIV screening. The authors reported that fear was a big factor for declining testing. The women are afraid to find out they are HIV-infected. They are frightened to discover a partner's infidelity. They are fearful of being judged by their health care provider or of being denied medical care if they tested positive (Rothpletz-Puglia et al, 2001).

Lancioni et al. reported that HIV-infected women did not participate in prenatal care because they fear disclosing their status to their caretakers and being judged by them for continuing the pregnancy (Lancioni et al., 1999). In a recent report by Lindau et al, HIV-infected women who were interviewed were aware of the benefits of prophylaxis treatment yet most received insufficient or no prenatal care. They knew of their HIV infection diagnosis but most did not disclose their status to their caretaker when they presented for delivery at hospitals capable of providing prophylaxis treatment. They attributed health care providers' lack of sensitivity, violations of confidentiality, disdain for HIV infection and substance abuse as reasons for their non-participation in prenatal care, avoidance of treatment for HIV infection, and non-disclosure of their HIV status. Denial and fear were other barriers to HIV prophylaxis treatment (Lindau, 2006).

We agreed with Lindau et al that may be what is needed to further reduce perinatal transmission beyond the conventional models for prevention is to understand the HIV-infected women's point of view, their fears and concerns and to eliminate the disrespect treatment as perceived by them from the health care providers. It is hope that we can create a medical environment where these women will be confident of our compassion and care to disclose their status and to want to seek prenatal care and HIV prophylaxis treatment (Lindau, 2006).

Lastly, not only obstetricians and gynecologists need to follow the CDC and ACOG guidelines in providing opt-out prenatal screening for HIV they must receive appropriate training for pre and post screening counseling and must ensure patient confidentiality. More importantly, at every screening they must be prepared for positive results: they must be compassionate toward those tested positive and must have resources available for their emotional support beyond providing the standard medical interventions to decrease vertical transmission.

Author details

Chi Dola*, Maga Martinez, Olivia Chang and Amanda Johnson

*Address all correspondence to: cdola@tulane.edu

Department of Obstetrics and Gynecology, Tulane University School of Medicine, New Orleans, Louisiana, USA

References

[1] Allen, V. M, Connell, O, Liston, C. M, & Baskett, R. M. T.F. ((2003). Maternal morbidity associated with cesarean deliverywithout labor compared with spontaneous onset of labor at term. Obstet Gynecol 2003; , 102, 477-82.

[2] American College of Obstetricians and Gynecologists. ACOG Committee Opinion Routine Human Immunodeficiency Virus Screening. Obstetrics and Gynecology (2008). , 112: 401-403.(411)

[3] American College of Obstetricians and Gynecologists. ACOG Committee Opinion Prenatal and Perinatal Human Immunodeficiency Virus Testing: Expanded Recommendations. Obstetrics and Gynecology (2008). , 112: 739-742.(418)

[4] American College of Obstetricians and GynecologistsACOG committee opinion # 234. Scheduled cesarean delivery and the prevention of vertical transmission of HIV infection. May, (2000).

[5] Bardeguez, A. D, Shapiro, D. E, Mofenson, L. M, Coombs, R, Frenkel, L. M, Fowler, M. G, et al. Effect of cessation of zidovudine prophylaxis to reduce vertical transmission on maternal HIV disease progression and survival. J Acquir Immune Defic Syndr (2003). , 32, 170-81.

[6] Brabin, L. (2002). Interactions of the Female Hormonal Environment, Susceptibility to Viral Infections, and Disease Progression. *AIDS Patient Care and STDs*, 211 EOF-221 EOF.

[7] Branson, B. M, Handsfield, H. H, Lampe, M. A, Janssen, R. S, Taylor, A. W, Lyss, S. B, & Clark, J. E. Revised Recommendations for HIV Testing of Adults, Adolescents, and Pregnant Women in Health-Care Settings. MMWR Recommendations and Reports (2006).

[8] Bulterys, M, Jamieson, D. J, Sullivan, O, Cohen, M. J, Maupin, M. H, & Nesheim, R. S. et al. Rapid HIV-1 testing during labor: a multicenter study. JAMA. (2004). , 292219-23.

[9] Centers for Disease Control and PreventionDiagnoses of HIV infection and AIDS in the United States and dependent areas, (2010). HIV Surveillance Report. Atlanta (GA): CDC; 2012. Available at: http://www.cdc.gov/hiv/surveillance/resources/ reports/2010report/pdf/2010_HIV_Surveillance_Report_pdf.Retrieved June 1, 2012.

[10] Centers for Disease Control and PreventionHIV/AIDS and women. Available at: http://www.cdc.gov/hiv/topics/women/overview_partner.htm.Retrieved June 29, (2012).

[11] Centers for Disease Control and PreventionHIV among women. Atlanta (GA): CDC; (2011). Available at: http://www.cdc.gov/hiv/topics/women/pdf/ women.pdf.Retrieved June 1, 2012.

[12] Centers for Disease Control and PreventionHIV surveillance-United States, 1981-2008. MMWR. (2011). , 2011, 60-689.

[13] Centers for Disease Control and PreventionMother-to-Child (Perinatal) HIV Trans-mission and Prevention. CDC HIV/AIDS Fact Sheet (2007).

[14] Centers for Disease Control and PreventionPediatric HIV Surveillance. http:// www.cdc.gov/hiv/topics/surveillance/resources/slides/pediatric.Accessed August 2, (2012).

[15] Centers for Disease Control and PreventionEstimated lifetime risk for diagnosis of HIV infection among Hispanics/Latinos-37 states and Puerto Rico, (2007). MMWR. , 59(40), 1297-1301.

[16] Centers for Disease Control and PreventionPublic Health Service Task Force recom-mendations for the use of antiretroviral drugs in pregnant women infected with HIV-1 for maternal health and for reducing perinatal HIV-1 transmission in the Unit-ed States. MMWR (1998). (RR-2)

[17] Chou, R, Smits, A. K, Huffman, L. H, Fu, R, & Korthuis, P. T. US Preventive Services Task Force. Prenatal screening for HIV: A review of the evidence for the U.S. Preven-tive Services Task Force. Ann Intern Med. (2005). Jul 5;, 143(1), 38-54.

[18] Coll, O, Fiore, S, Floridia, M, et al. (2002). Pregnancy and HIV infection: a European consensus on management. AIDS, 2002; 16(suppl):S, 1-18.

[19] Connor, E. M, Sperling, R. S, Gelber, R, Kiselev, P, Scott, G, & Sullivan, O. MJ, et al. Reduction of maternal-infant transmission of human immunodeficiency virus type 1

with zidovudine treatment. Pediatric AIDS Clinical Trials Group Protocol 076 Study Group. N Engl J Med (1994). , 331, 1173-80.

[20] Cooper, E. R, Charurat, M, Mofenson, L, Hanson, I. C, Pitt, J, Diaz, C, et al. Combination antiretroviral strategies for the treatment of pregnant HIV-1-infected women and prevention of perinatal HIV-1 transmission. J Acquir Immune Defic Syndr (2002). , 29, 484-94.

[21] Dabis, F, Msellati, P, Meda, N, Welffens-ekra, C, You, B, Manigart, O, et al. month efficacy, tolerance, and acceptability of a short regimen of oral zidovudine to reduce vertical transmission of HIV in breastfed children in Cote d'Ivoire and Burkina Faso: a double-blind placebo-controlled multicentre trial. DITRAME Study Group. Diminution de la Transmission Mere-Enfant. Lancet (1999). , 353, 786-92.

[22] De Cock, K. M, Fowler, M. G, Mercier, E, et al. (2000). Prevention of Mother-to-child HIV transmission in resource-poor countries: translating research into policy and practice. JAMA. 283(9).

[23] Determinants of mother-to-infant human immunodeficiency virus 1 transmission before and after the introduction of zidovudine prophylaxisArch Pediatr Adolesc Med (2002). , 156, 915-21.

[24] Dunn, D. T, Newell, M. L, Ades, A. E, & Peckham, C. S. Risk of human immunodeficiency virus type 1 transmission through breastfeeding. Lancet. (1992). , 340585-8.

[25] Efficacy of three short-course regimens of zidovudine and lamivudine in preventing early and late transmission of HIV-1 from mother to child in TanzaniaSouth Africa, and Uganda (Petra study): a randomised, double-blind, placebo-controlled trial. Lancet (2002). , 359, 1178-86.

[26] European collaborative study and the Swiss Mother + Child HIV Cohort Study ((2000). Combination antiretroviral therapy andduration of pregnancy. AIDS. 2000;, 14, 2913-20.

[27] Gray, R. H, Li, X, Kigazi, G, Serwadda, D, Brahmbhatt, H, Wabwire-mangen, F, Nalugoda, F, Kiddugavu, M, Sweankambo, N, Quinn, T. C, Reynolds, S. J, & Wawer, M. J. Increased Risk of Incident HIV during Pregnancy in Rakai, Uganda: A Prospective Study. The Lancet (2005).

[28] Grubert, T. A, Reindell, D, Belohradsky, B. H, Gurtler, L, Stauber, M, & Dathe, O. Rates of postoperative complication among human immunodeficiency virus-infected women who have undergone obstetric and gynecologic surgical procedures. CID (2002). , 34, 822-30.

[29] Grosch-woerner, I, Puch, K, Maier, R. F, Niehues, T, Notheis, G, Patel, D, et al. Multicenter Interdisciplinary Study GroupGermany/Austria. Increased rate of prematurity associated with antenatal antiretroviral therapy in a German/Austrian cohort ofHIV-1-infected women. HIV Med. (2008). , 9, 6-13.

[30] Guay, L. A, Musoke, P, Fleming, T, Bagenda, D, Allen, M, Nakabiito, C, et al. Intra-partum and neonatal single-dose nevirapine compared with zidovudine for preven-tion of mother-to-child transmission of HIV-1 in Kampala, Uganda: HIVNET 012 randomised trial. Lancet (1999). , 354, 795-802.

[31] Hall, H. I, An, Q, Hutchinson, A. B, & Sansom, S. Estimating the lifetime risk of a di-agnosis of the HIV infection in 33 states, (2004). J Acquir Immune Defic Syndr 2008;, 49, 294-7.

[32] Holtgrave, D. R, Hall, H. I, Rhodes, P. H, et al. (2009). Updated annual HIV transmis-sion rates in the United States, 1977-2006. J Acquir Immune Defic Syndr , 50(2), 236-238.

[33] Grubert, T. A, Reindell, D, Kastner, R, Lutz-friedrich, R, Belohradsky, B. H, & Datha, O. Complications after caesarean section in HIV-1 infected women not taking antire-troviral treatment. Lancet, (1999). , 354, 1612-3.

[34] Jamieson, D. J, Read, J. S, Kourtis, A. P, Durant, T. M, Lampe, M. A, & Dominguez, K. L. Cesarean delivery for HIV-infected women: recommendations and controversies. Am J Obstet Gynecol. (2007). Sep;197(3 Suppl):S, 96-100.

[35] John, G. C, Richardson, B. A, Nduati, R. W, Mbori-ngacha, D, & Kreiss, J. K. Timing of breast milk HIV-1 transmission: a meta-analysis.. East Afr Med J. (2001). , 7875-9.

[36] Koenig, L. J, Whitaker, D. J, Royce, R. A, Wilson, T. E, Callahan, M. R, Fernandez, M. I, et al. Violence during pregnancy among women with or at risk for HIV infection.. Am J Public Health. (2002). , 92367-70.

[37] Kourtis, A. P, Lee, F. K, Abrams, E. J, et al. Mother-to-child transmission of HIV-1: timing and implications for prevention. Lancet Infect Dis. (2006). , 6, 726-732.

[38] Lancioni, C, Harwell, T, & Rutstein, R. M. (1999). Prenatal care and HIV infection. AIDS Patient Care STDS. 1999 Feb; 13 (2); , 97-102.

[39] Lallemant, M, & Jourdain, G. Le Coeur S, Kim S, Koetsawang S, Comeau AM, et al. A trial of shortened zidovudine regimens to prevent mother-to-child transmission of human immunodeficiency virus type 1. Perinatal HIV Prevention Trial (Thailand) In-vestigators. N Engl J Med (2000). , 343, 982-91.

[40] Lester, P, Partridge, J. C, Chesney, M. A, & Cooke, M. The consequences of a positive prenatal HIV antibody test for women. J Acquir Immune Defic Syndr Hum Retrovir-ol. (1995). , 10341-9.

[41] Lindau, S, Jerome, J, Miller, K, Monk, E, Garcia, P, & Cohen, M. (2006). Mothers on the margins: Implications for eradicating perinatal HIV. Social Science and Medicine, 62(1), 59-69.

[42] Livingston, E, Huo, Y, Patel, K, Brogly, S. B, Tuomala, R, Scott, G. B, Bardeguez, A, Stek, A, & Read, J. S. (2010). For the International Maternal Pediatric Adolescent AIDS Clinical Trials Group (IMPAACT) Protocol 1025 Study. Mode of Delivery and

Infant Respiratory Morbidity Among Infants Born to HIV-1 infected Women. Obstet Gynecol, 2010; 116(2 Pt 1): 335-343.

[43] Makoha, F. W, Felimban, H. M, Fathuddien, M. A, Roomi, F, & Ghabra, T. (2004). Multiple cesarean section morbidity. Int J Gynaecol Obstet 2004; , 87, 227-32.

[44] Mandelbrot, L, Landreau-mascaro, A, Rekacewicz, C, Berrebi, A, Benifla, J. L, Burgard, M, et al. Lamivudine-zidovudine combination for prevention of maternal-infant transmission of HIV-1. JAMA (2001). , 285, 2083-93.

[45] Marks, G, Crepaz, N, & Janssen, R. (2006). Estimating sexual transmission of HIV from persons aware and unaware that they are infected with the virus in the USA. Journal of Acquired Immune Deficiency Sydromes , 20(10), 1447-1450.

[46] Minkoff, H, Mccalla, S, & Feldman, J. (1990). The relationship of cocaine use to syphilis and HIV infection among inner city parturient women. Am J Obstet Gynecol. 1990;, 163, 521-526.

[47] Moodley, D, Moodley, J, Coovadia, H, Gray, G, Mcintyre, J, Hofmyer, J, et al. A multicenter randomized, controlled trial of nevirapine versus a combination of zidovudine and lamivudine to reduce intrapartum and early postpartum mother-to-child transmission of human immunodeficiency virus type 1. J Infect Dis (2003). , 187, 725-35.

[48] Moodley, D, Esterhuizen, T. M, Pather, T, Chetty, V, & Ngaleka, L. High HIV Incidence During Pregnancy: Compelling Reason for Repeat HIV Testing. AIDS (2009).

[49] Mother-to-child transmission of HIV infection in the era of highly active antiretroviral therapyClin Infect Dis (2005). , 40, 458-65.

[50] Nduati, R, John, G, Mbori-ngacha, D, Richardson, B, Overbaugh, J, Mwatha, A, et al. Effect of breastfeeding and formula feeding on transmission of HIV-1: a randomized clinical trial.. JAMA. (2000). , 2831167-74.

[51] Provisional Committee on Pediatric AIDSAmerican Academy of Pediatrics. Perinatal human immunodeficiency virus testing. Pediatrics. (1995). , 95303-7.

[52] Prejean, J, Song, R, Hernandez, A, Ziebell, R, Green, T, et al. Estimated HIV Incidence in the United States, (2011). PLoS ONE 2011 6(8): e17502. doi:10.1371/journal.pone. 0017502., 2006-2009.

[53] Public Health Service Task Force(2010). Recommendations for use of antiretroviral drugs in pregnant HIV-infected women for maternal health and interventions to reduce perinatal HIV-1 transmission in the United States. 2010. Available at: http:// aidsinfo.nih.gov/contentfiles/PerinatalGL.pdfRetrieved April 13, 2011., 1.

[54] Rahangdale, L, & Cohan, D. Rapid Human Immunodeficiency Virus Testing on Labor and Delivery. Obstetrics and Gynecology (2008).

[55] Read, J. S, Tuomala, R, Kpamegan, E, Zorrilla, C, Landesman, S, Brown, G, et al. Mode of delivery and postpartum morbidity among HIV-infected women: the women and infants transmission study. J Acquir Immune Defic Syndr (2001). , 26, 236-45.

[56] Rothpletz-puglia, P, Storm, D, Burr, C, & Samuels, D. Routine prenatal HIV testing: women's concern and their strategies for addressing concerns. Matern Child Health J (2012).

[57] Samson, L, & King, S. Evidence-based guidelines for universal counselling and offering of HIV testing in pregnancy in Canada.. CMAJ. (1998). , 1581449-57.

[58] Sansom, S. L, Jamieson, D. J, Farnham, P. G, Bulterys, M, & Fowler, M. G. Human Immunodeficiency Virus Retesting During Pregnancy: Costs and Effectiveness in Preventing Perinatal Transmission. Obstetrics and Gynecology (2003).

[59] Shaffer, N, Chuachoowong, R, Mock, P. A, Bhadrakom, C, Siriwasin, W, Young, N. L, et al. Short-course zidovudine for perinatal HIV-1 transmission in Bangkok, Thailand: a randomised controlled trial. Bangkok Collaborative Perinatal HIV Transmission Study Group. Lancet (1999). , 353, 773-80.

[60] Sheon, A. R, Fox, H. E, Alexander, G, Buck, A, Higgins, A, Mcdermott, S. M, et al. Misdiagnosed HIV infection in pregnant women: implications for clinical care.. Public Health Rep. (1994). , 109694-9.

[61] Shernoff, M, & Smith, R. HIV treatments: A history of scientific advance. Body Positive Magazine. July (2001).

[62] Sturt, A. S, Dokubo, E. K, & Sint, T. T. Antiretroviral therapy (ART) for treating HIV infection in ART-eligible pregnant women. Cochrane Database of Systematic Reviews (2010). Issue 3. Art. DOI:CD008440.(CD008440)

[63] Taha, T. E, Kumwenda, N. I, Gibbons, A, Broadhead, R. L, Fiscus, S, Lema, V, et al. Short postexposure prophylaxis in newborn babies to reduce mother-to-child transmission of HIV-1: NVAZ randomised clinical trial. Lancet (2003). , 362, 1171-7.

[64] Tita, A. T, Landon, M. B, Spong, C. Y, Lai, Y, Leveno, K. J, Varner, M. W, Moawad, A. H, Caritis, S. N, Meis, P. J, Wapner, R. J, Sorokin, Y, Miodovnik, M, Carpenter, M, Peaceman, A. M, Sullivan, O, Sibai, M. J, Langer, B. M, Thorp, O, Ramin, J. M, & Mercer, S. M. B.M.; Eunice Kennedy Shriver NICHD Maternal-Fetal Medicine Units Network. Timing of elective repeat cesarean delivery at term and neonatal outcomes. N Engl J Med, (2009). , 360(2), 111-20.

[65] The International Perinatal HIV GroupThe mode of delivery and the risk for vertical transmission of human immunodeficiency virus type a meta-analysis of 15 prospective cohort studies. N Engl J Med. (1999). , 1.

[66] Turner, B. J, Mckee, L. J, Siverman, N. S, et al. (1996). Prenatal care and birth outcomes of a cohort of HIV-infected women. J Acquir Immune Defic Syndr 1996; , 12, 259-67.

[67] UNFPA/UNICEF/WHO/UNAIDS Inter-Agency Task Team on Mother-to-Child Transmission of HIVNew data on the prevention of mother-to-child transmission of HIV and their policy implications: conclusions and recommendations. Geneva, Switzerland: World Health Organization; (2000).

[68] Vimercati, A, Greco, P, Loverro, G, Lopalco, P. L, Pansini, V, & Selvaggi, L. (2000). Maternal complications after caesarean section in HIV infected women. Eur J Obstet Gynecol Reprod Biol, 2000;, 90, 73-76.

[69] Watts, D. H, Lambert, J. S, Stiehm, E. R, Bethel, J, Whitehouse, J, Fowler, M. G, et al. Complications according to mode of delivery among human immunodeficiency virus-infected women with CD4 lymphocyte counts of < or = 500/microL. Am J Obstet Gynecol (2000). , 183, 100-7.

[70] Watts, D. H, & Balasubramanian, R. Maupin RT Jr, Delke I, Dorenbaum A, Fiore S, et al. Maternal toxicity and pregnancy complications in human immunodeficiency virus-infected women receiving antiretroviral therapy: PACTG 316. Am J Obstet Gynecol (2004). , 190, 506-16.

[71] Wiktor, S. Z, Ekpini, E, Karon, J. M, Nkengasong, J, Maurice, C, Severin, S. T, et al. Short-course oral zidovudine for prevention of mother-to-child transmission of HIV-1 in Abidjan, Cote d'Ivoire: a randomised trial. Lancet (1999). , 353, 781-5.

Chapter 5

Human Immunodeficiency Virus Testing Algorithm in Resource Limiting Settings

Teddy Charles Adias and Osaro Erhabor

Additional information is available at the end of the chapter

1. Introduction

Testing and counseling for human immunodeficiency virus (HIV) is now recognized as a priority in national HIV programs because it is the gateway to HIV/AIDS prevention, care, treatment, and support interventions. In order to ensure access to HIV testing for large populations and to facilitate access to antiretroviral treatment in the context of the World Health Organization's universal access strategy, radical scaling up of HIV testing and counseling services is being advocated globally.

The use of HIV rapid tests will facilitate this in many settings, particularly in services in which the people most likely to benefit from knowing their HIV status can be reached. These Settings include diagnostic and treatment services for tuberculosis and sexually transmitted infections; services linked to the prevention of mother-to-child transmission of HIV; the management of occupational and non-occupational exposures to HIV; at voluntary counseling and testing (VCT) sites; in remote areas where the creation and maintenance of a laboratory infrastructure is not possible; and where hard-to-reach populations have access to HIV testing (PAHO, 2008).

To date, HIV testing strategies has clear objective for diagnosis, surveillance and transfusion safety. The need for appropriate selection of testing platforms and protocol had also varied from setting to setting. In general, four criteria had underpinned the choice of most appropriate test or combination of tests for any given setting and depend on: General goal for testing, Diagnostic indices of sensitivity and specificity, Prevalence of HIV infection in the general population and Cost of testing (WHO, 2004).

HIV testing is the entry point for both care and prevention. In resource limiting settings, this declaration seems more valid than ever given the increase prevalence and incidence of HIV infection in these settings and current efforts at universal access for care and prevention. The aim of this chapter is to provide trend in HIV testing Algorithm- a combination and sequence of specific testing employed in given strategy for the confirmation of HIV status of an individual or sample.

In the evolving Chapter, we shall transit with set-out for HIV testing algorithms (with appropriate sub-themes) from HIV testing evolution and forms of testing to HIV testing strategies and algorithm platforms.

2. HIV testing

2.1. Evolution of HIV testing

HIV screening and diagnostic tests have been developed, and a variety of testing algorithms have come into use. HIV antibody tests have evolved from first generation HIV-1(clade B) viral lysate-based, indirect antibody enzyme immunoassays (EIAs) to third generation antigen-sandwich immunoassays that use synthetic peptide and recombinant DNA derived antigens that represent the immunodominant epitopes from diverse HIV-1 and HIV-2 strains. These third generation enzyme immunoassays have substantially enhanced sensitivity to divergent viral variants and have shortened the infection-to-seroconversion window period by more than 3 weeks compared with first generation tests. Assays have also been developed that detect and quantitate viral antigen (p24) and nucleic acids (HIV RNA or DNA) in blood, and in body fluids and tissues (Branson, 2010; WHO, 2009a).

These assays have seen increasing application in blood and organ donor screening, as well as in clinical diagnosis, prognosis, and therapeutic monitoring; and clinicians now have access to a broad and potentially confusing array of test options, each with its own advantages and limitations. Developing testing algorithms and interpretive criteria appropriate to a particular group of patients—high-risk adults; blood, plasma and organ donors; recently exposed healthcare workers; paediatric patients, and especially in resource limiting settings—poses a challenge, especially as new tests appear with tantalizing claims of enhanced performance (WHO, 2009a/b).

The laboratory diagnosis of the HIV infection is based on a two-stage strategy: a screening analysis followed by a confirmation analysis. A positive screening analysis must always be supplemented by a confirmation analysis on the same sample. An HIV infection can only be confirmed when the result of the confirmation analysis is positive and consistent results are obtained for two separate samples (PAHO, 2008).

Screening tests provide presumptive identification of specimens that contain antibody to HIV. These enzyme immunosorbent assays (EIAs) or simple/rapid immuno-diagnostics are selected for their high sensitivity of detecting antibodies to HIV. Supplemental or confirmatory tests, such as Western blot (WB), can be used to confirm infection in samples that are initially reactive on conventional EIAs. Alternatively, repetitive testing incorporating EIAs or rapid tests selected for their specificity may be used to confirm whether specimens found to be reactive for HIV antibodies with a particular screening test are specific to HIV. For practical purposes, resource-poor settings depend heavily on EIA and rapid tests for screening and confirmation (WHO, 2004).

2.2. Enzyme immunsorbent assays

EIAs are the most widely used screening tests because of their suitability for analyzing large numbers of specimens, particularly in blood screening centers. Since 1985, EIAs have progressed considerably from first to fourth generation assays: first generation assays were based on purified HIV whole viral lysates, however, sensitivity and specificity of these assays were poor; second generation assays used HIV-recombinant proteins and/or synthetic peptides, which enabled the production of assays capable of detecting HIV-1 and HIV-2. The assays had improved specificity, although their overall sensitivity was similar to that of first-generation assays. Third-generation assays used the solid phase coated with recombinant antigens and /or peptides and similar recombinant antigens and peptides conjugated to a detection enzyme or hapten that could detect HIV-specific antibodies bound to a solid phase. These assays could detect immunoglobulin M, early antibodies to HIV, in addition to IgG, thus resulting in a reduction of the seroconversion window. Fourth generation assays are very similar to third-generations tests but have the ability to detect simultaneously HIV antibodies and antigens. Typical fourth-generation EIAs incorporate cocktails of HIV-1 group M (HIV-1 p24, HIV-1 gp160), HIV-1 group O, and HIV-2 antigens (HIV-2 env peptide) (WHO, 2009a/b and 2004).

Furthermore, third and fourth-generation assays are able to detect IgM and IgG antibodies to both HIV-1 and HIV-2. These assays may reduce the 2-4 week time period, "window period" of detecting HIV antibodies (WHO, 2009b).

2.3. Rapid/simple assays

Simple, instrument-free assays are also available and are now widely used in Africa. They include agglutination, immunofiltration, and immunochromatographic assays. The appearance of a colored dot or line, or an agglutination pattern indicates a positive result. Most of these tests can be performed in less than 20 minutes, and are therefore called simple/rapid assays. Some simple tests, such as agglutination assays, are less rapid and may require about 30 minutes to 2 hours to be completed. In general, these rapid/simple tests are most suitable for use in settings that have limited facilities and process fewer than 100 samples per day (WHO, 2009b and 2004).

2.3.1. Importance of rapid/simple assays

Although EIA–based serodiagnostic algorithms are highly cost effective, their application in resource-poor settings is limited by several factors. They require well-trained personnel, need a consistent supply of electricity, and maintenance and cost of most equipment. Rapid assays have high sensitivity and specificity and perform as well as EIAs on specimens from persons seroconverting for non-B HIV-1 subtypes (Koblavi-Dème *et al*, 2001). Rapid enzyme assays circumvent the issue of low rates of return for serologic results associated with EIA-based testing algorithms because results can be delivered on the same day (Puro *et al*, 2004). In addition, their performance has improved considerably, and some do not require recon-stitution of reagents or refrigeration; thus, making them very suitable for use in resource limited settings and hard to reach populations (Koblavi-Dème *et al*, 2001). Practical applica-tions for the use of simple/rapid assays are in settings such as Voluntary Counseling and Testing (VCT) and Prevention of Mother to Child Transmission (PMTCT) programs. Studies have shown that using rapid assay testing algorithms result in remarkable increase in the number of HIV-positive women identified as eligible to receive the short-course therapy that reduces mother-to-child transmission of HIV (Sibailly *et al*, 2000).

3. HIV testing strategies and algorithm

3.1. Nature of algorithm/testing strategy

A testing algorithm for serologic diagnosis of HIV-infection is the sequence in which assays are performed to detect HIV antibody in a body fluid. The most common referenced testing algorithm employs an EIA to screen specimens with those found to be positive then con-firmed by WB testing. This so-called conventional algorithm has several limitations (PAHO, 2008):

- WB is expensive and requires technical expertise.

- WB often yields indeterminate results with certain types of specimens with uncertain di-agnostic significance, e.g., hyperimmunoglobulinemia specimens.

- Both ELISA and WB are time consuming and require a well-equipped laboratory infra-structure.

Various combinations of tests can be used: combinations of HIV EIAs; combinations of rapid tests; or an EIA in conjunction with rapid tests. The choice of strategy and of HIV tests should be determined by the quality of the tests and by the practicality of their implementa-tion, logistics, and the cost-benefit analysis. Figure 1, depicts the WHO/UNAIDS testing strategies which can be adopted in diverse settings

In the WHO/UNAIDS testing strategies I – III, as applicable relative to testing objective (sur-veillance, blood screening, or diagnosis) or diagnostic indices (sero-prevalence in a given population and the duo of sensitivity and specificity of the test being used. The three HIV testing strategies recommended by WHO and UNAIDS are described below (Figure 1) (WHO, 2009a; UNAID/WHO, 1998).

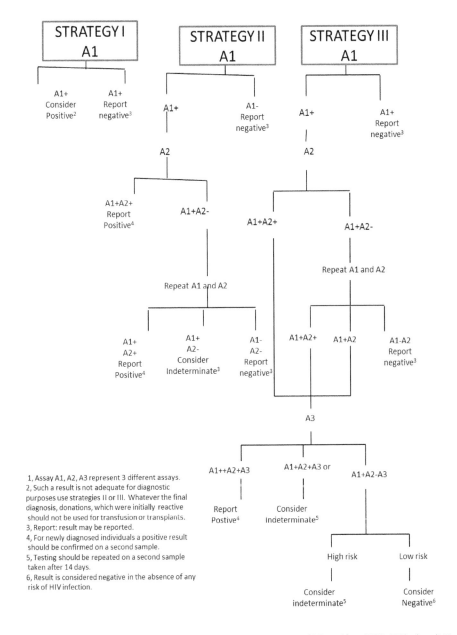

Figure 1. Schematic Representation of the WHO/UNAIDS HIV Testing Strategy(Adapted from WHO, 2009a/b and UN-AID/WHO,1998)

Strategy I:

• Requires one test.

• For use in diagnostic testing in populations with an HIV prevalence >30% among persons with clinical signs or symptoms of HIV infection.

• For use in blood screening, for all prevalence rates.

• For use in surveillance testing in populations with an HIV prevalence >10% (example: un-linked anonymous testing for surveillance among pregnant women at antenatal clinics). No results are provided.

Strategy II:

• Requires up to two tests.

• For use in diagnostic testing in populations with an HIV prevalence ≤30% among persons with clinical signs or symptoms of HIV infection or >10% among asymptomatic persons.

• For use in surveillance testing in populations with an HIV prevalence ≤10% (example: un-linked anonymous testing for surveillance among patients at antenatal clinics or sexually transmitted infection clinics). No results are provided.

Strategy III:

• Requires up to three tests.

• For use in diagnostic testing in populations with an HIV prevalence ≤10% among asymp-tomatic persons.

Sensitivity and specificity are two important factors that determine a test's accuracy in distinguishing between HIV-infected and uninfected individuals. It is crucial that the HIV tests used in the algorithms all have a sensitivity of at least 99% and a specificity of at least 98% (WHO, 2009a and 1997). There are commercially available HIV EIAs and HIV rapid tests that meet these criteria. When selecting HIV tests to be used in combination, it is important to select tests that do not share the same false positive and same false negative results. This information can be obtained from comparative evaluation studies of HIV test kits, such as those published in international scientific publications and in WHO reports (WHO, 2009a/b). It is recommended that such comparative evaluations of a select number of HIV test kits be conducted at the national and/or regional level prior to the establishment of the national HIV test algorithms. These principles apply to both conventional HIV EIA and HIV rapid tests. The national reference laboratory should validate a select number of test kits for use in the national HIV testing algorithms.

Specific implementation requirements must be considered when selecting tests kits and al-gorithms. For example, will testing be performed in a laboratory setting, or in a VCT or clini-cal setting without extensive laboratory facilities? In settings without extensive laboratory facilities or where clients do not return for follow-up visits, algorithms using only rapid tests are preferred. In situations in which patients return at regular intervals (e.g., TB clinics) or in prenatal clinics where blood specimens are taken for other testing purposes, the set-up may allow for HIV EIA-based algorithms or algorithms combining EIA and rapid tests (Owusu-Ofori et al, 2005; Routet et al, 2004).

Another factor determining the most cost-efficient approach is the volume of specimens to be processed daily or weekly. An EIA test is half the price of a rapid test, so if a particular setting processes 40 specimens a day and the laboratory has the required equipment, it is more cost effective to use EIAs than rapid tests. It is important that the HIV tests and algorithms be chosen carefully and with the aim of optimal integration into the existing health care facilities, minimizing the potential to disrupt their operations or unnecessarily overburden staff.

There are many strategies for HIV testing (Parekh *et al*, 2010; WHO, 2009a/b; P*aul et al, 2004*). WHO, CDC, and the Association of Public Health Laboratories have jointly developed one of the most useful references for HIV testing algorithms. These strategies can be divided into two approaches: serial (or sequential) testing and parallel testing.

3.2. Algorithm platforms

3.2.1. Serial/sequential testing strategy

In a Serial or sequential testing strategy, samples are initially tested with only one, highly sensitive assay. Samples that are reactive in the first assay are then re-tested using a second, highly specific assay. A third test may be performed, depending on the result of the second assay and the objective of the testing. Both the selection of and the order in which the assays are used are of the utmost importance for the final outcome of the tests. If test combinations are not carefully selected, individuals may be incorrectly diagnosed. WHO recommends sequential testing (Figure 2) in most settings because it is more economical, as the second test is required only when the initial test result is positive (Gershy=Damet *et al*, 2010; WHO, 2009a/b; Ferreira *et al*, 2005).

3.2.2. Parallel testing strategy

In a parallel testing strategy (Figure 3), samples are tested using two different assays simultaneously. This approach is rather expensive, as it virtually doubles the cost of testing in low- prevalence settings by requiring two tests at the outset. As with sequential testing, a third test may be performed preferably at the secondary level, where laboratory facilities and experienced staff are available, depending on the result of the assays and the objective of the testing (WHO, 2009a/b).

Therefore, the parallel testing strategy is recommended only in situations in which it can add value. Prenatal clinics provide one such example: A woman's first visit to the clinic may be to deliver her child, thus requiring a rapid decision whether an intervention to prevent mother-to-child transmission of HIV is needed. Other emergency situations, such as work accidents, sexual violence, and discordant couples also would benefit from this strategy. In these cases, two rapid tests using whole-blood finger-stick specimens in parallel will pro-

vide the answer in just 10–15 minutes. HIV rapid tests using wholeblood finger-stick specimens have great potential in situations where results need to be known quickly, or where
taking a conventional venous sample is difficult (Gershy-Damet *et al*, 2010; WHO, 2009a/b;
Ferreira *et al*, 2005).

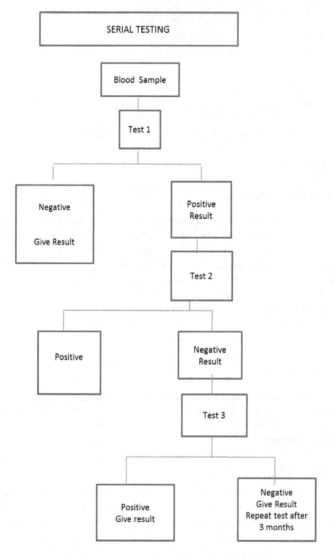

Figure 2. Serial/ Sequential Testing Algorithm (Adapted from WHO, 2009a/b)

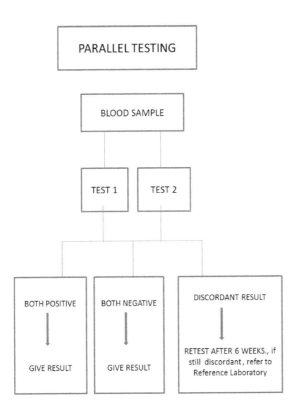

Figure 3. Parallel Testing Algorithm (Adapted from WHO, 2009a/b)

4. Conclusion

HIV testing is the essential entry point for both treatment and prevention. As in all societies, especially in Africa, high degree of genetic diversity exist. One implication for this is the need for each country to have an in-house evaluation of its country –specific testing strategy. The selection of a national algorithm is the responsibility of the country's Ministry of Health. The choice of sequential or parallel testing should be made after a thorough analysis of the scientific evidence, logistics, test performance requirements, and cost/affordability of the various algorithms.

Author details

Teddy Charles Adias[1*] and Osaro Erhabor[2]

*Address all correspondence to: teddyadias@yahoo.com

1 Bayelsa State College of Health Technology, Ogbia Town, Yenagoa, Nigeria

2 Department of Blood Sciences, Royal Bolton Hospital NHS Trust UK, Bolton, United Kingdom

References

[1] Branson BM (2010). The future of HIV testing. *JAIDS.* 55 (2): 102-105.

[2] Ferreira Junior OC, Ferreira C, Riedel M, Widolin MR, Barbosa-Júnior A (2005). HIV Rapid Test Study Group.Evaluation of rapid tests for anti-HIV detection in Brazil. *AIDS.*19(4):S70–75.

[3] Gershy-Damet G, Rotz P, Cross, D, *et al* (2010). The World Health Organization African region laboratory accreditation process: Improving the quality of laboratory systems in the African region. *Am J Clin Pathol. 134* : 393-400.

[4] Koblavi-Dème S, Maurice C, Yavo D, *et al* (2001). Sensitivity and specificity of HIV rapid serologic assays and testing algorithms in an antenatal clinic in Abidjan, Côte d'Ivoire. *J Clin Microbiol.* 39:1808-1812.

[5] Owusu-Ofori S, Temple J, Sarkodie F, Anokwa M, Candotti D, Allain JP (2005). Predonation screening of blood donors with rapid tests: Implementation and efficacy of a novel approach to blood safety in resource-poor settings. *Transfusion.* 45(2):133–140.

[6] Pan American Health Organisation (PAHO) (2008). Guidelines for the implementation of Reliable and Efficient Diagnostic HIV Testing, Region of the Americas.

[7] Parekh B, Kalou M, Alemnji G, Ou C, *et al* (2010). Scaling up HIV rapid testing in developing countries: comprehensive approach for implementing quality assurance. *Am J Clin Pathol.* 134: 573-84.

[8] Paul SM, Grimes-Dennis J, Burr CK, DiFerdinando GT (2003). Rapid diagnostic testing for HIV. Clinical implications. *N J Med* 100(9):11–14.

[9] Puro V, Francisci D, Sighinolfi L, Civljak R, Belfiori B, Deparis P, et al (2004) Benefits of a rapid HIV test for evaluation of the source patient after occupational exposure of healthcare workers. *J Hosp Infect.* 57(2):179–182.

[10] Rouet F, Ekouevi DK, Inwoley A, Chaix ML, Burgard M, Bequet L, et al (2004). Field evaluation of a rapid human immunodeficiency virus (HIV) serial serologic testing

algorithm for diagnosis and differentiation of HIV type 1 (HIV-1), HIV-2, and dual HIV-1–HIV-2 infections in West African pregnant women. *J Clin Microbiol.* 42(9): 4147–4153.

[11] Sibailly TS, Ekpini ER, Kamelan-Tanoh A, *et al* (2000). Impact of on-site HIV rapid testing with same-day post-test counseling on acceptance of short-course zidovudine for the prevention of mother-to-child transmission of HIV in Abidjan, Côte d'Ivoire. *The XIII International AIDS 2000 Conference.*

[12] UNAIDS/WHO (1998). UNAIDS/WHO Recommendations. The importance of simple/rapid assays in HIV testing. Weekly Epidemiological Record. 73:321-28.

[13] World Health Organisation (WHO) (2009a). *HIV assays. Operational characteristics.* Report 16. *Rapid assay.* Geneva.

[14] World Health Organisation (WHO) (2009b). Guidelines for using HIV testing technologies in surveillance: Selection, Evaluation and Implementation 2009 Update

[15] World Health Organisation (WHO) (2004). Rapid HIV tests: guidelines for use in HIV testing and counseling services in resource-constrained settings.

[16] WHO/UNAIDS (1997). Revised Recommendations for the selection and use of HIV antibody tests. WHO Weekly Epidemiol. *72:* 81-7.

HIV and NeuroAIDS

Chapter 6

NeuroAIDS: Mechanisms, Causes, Prevalence, Diagnostics and Social Issues

Shailendra K. Saxena, Sneham Tiwari and
Madhavan P.N. Nair

Additional information is available at the end of the chapter

1. Introduction

Human immunodeficiency virus-1 (HIV-1) engulfs 33 millions of life as per the latest UN AIDS report [Saxena, Tiwari., *et al.*, 2012] and the effect worsens up when it causes dementia with alarming occurrence worldwide but the mechanism through which it happens is still not well understood, and is in the embryonic stages. The estimated overall prevalence of nervous system disorders among patients receiving highly active antiretroviral therapy but also requiring neurological care is over 25% (Singh *et al.*, 2011). According to WHO there are ~ 34 million people in the world infected with HIV. Out of that 95 percent of these cases as well as deaths from AIDS occur in the developing world. Dementia (HIV-associated dementia) is becoming common in HIV infected adults having prevalence up to 40% in western countries where clade B prevails (Sacktor *et al.*, 2007). Dementia cannot be considered as a disease by itself but it is the term used to describe a set of symptoms resulting from damages and disorders affecting the brain. These symptoms can be caused by a multitude of diseases and depend upon the specific brain regions affected. These symptoms appear as a variety of cognitive, behavioural, affective, motor, and psychiatric disorders. Dementia can be caused by a variety of diseases, known as neurodegenerative diseases resulting from protein aggregation in the brain. Many studies related to this area are been carried out in respect to this, to provide new insights (Saxena *et al.*, 2012). HIV-1 infects macrophages and microglia, and there is an indirect pathway to neuronal injury which happens due to release of macrophage, microglial and astrocytes toxins and viral proteins. The toxins which are released over stimulate neurons, form free radicals, finally leading to neurodegenerative diseases. The cognitive and motor dysfunction which is observed in HIV patients is termed as HIV associated dementia (HAD). The prevalence of the dementia is eventually increasing as AIDS patients are now surviving more. HIV-1 replicates in monocyte and macrophage but not as severe as in infected T cells and blood mononuclear cells (Sundaravaradan *et al.*, 2006). These cells differentiate and travel to several organs, henceforth acting as a source of infectious virus and secreted viral proteins to cause pathological issues and alternating several signalling pathways and distorting many cellular transcription factors, ultimately resulting in HIV-1 pathogenesis. Increased transcription leads to the upregulation of virus production, and hence increased production of viral proteins (gp120, Tat, Nef, and Vpr) (Gandhi et al., 2020; Samikkannu et al., 2010; Saiyed et al., 2011; Saxena et al., 2012; Saxena et al., 2012). The high concentration of these toxic proteins lead to distorted cellular functions, and increased production of toxic metabolites, finally leading to organ-specific like neuroAIDS, in case of viral entry inside the brain (Kilareski et al., 2009). Antiretroviral therapy has increased the lifespan of HIV patients, but CNS function often remains diminished sometimes developing into HIV-associated dementia and the severity and progression of dementia is studied to be increased with the effect of drug abuse [Reddy *et al.*, 2012; Ferris *et al.*, 2008].

2. Prevalence

The prevalence of HAD is estimated to be more than 30% of HIV infected patients, and it is still reported to be increasing (Dean *et al.*, 2012). Improvements in control of peripheral viral replication and the treatment of opportunistic infections, helps in extending life expectancy, resulting in an increase in neuropathogenesis. We are seeing a linear increase in prevalence in rich countries, but an exponential increase in low-income countries. Just under half of people with dementia live in high-income countries, 39% live in middle-income countries, and only 14% live in low-income countries. Increasing living standards, in low income countries such as India (Shankar *et al.*, 2005), may lead to increased life expectancy, which may increase the frequency of dementia cases. As biggest risk factor for dementia is age, a longer-living global population means there will be more people with dementia. The report predicts that the numbers of people with dementia will double every 20 years, to 65.7 million in 2030 and 115.4 million in 2050. Most of this increase will be in developing countries (Prince *et al.*, 2012). A more complete understanding of the pathogenesis of HAD will help in identifying therapeutic targets for its prevention and treatment. The global age standardized death rate for dementia is ~ 6.7 per 100,000 for males and 7.7 per 100,000 for females. According to the World Health Organization, dementia mortality rate for India is 13.5 per 100,000 males and 11.1 for 100,000 females, which is quite alarming (Prince *et al.*, 2012).

3. HIV- Mechanism of neuronal injury

Presently, neuropathogenesis is winning, because there is an incomplete knowledge about the mechanism of HIV infection causing neuronal injury and apoptosis in the host (Fig. 1). HIV enters the central nervous system through infected monocytes and leads to pathogenesis involving activation of macrophages and microglia and further toxin release, that activates several pathways leading to neuronal dysfunction. There are several extracellular and intracellular signalling pathways, which when activated lead to macrophage or microglial activation, and induction in neurons and astrocytes. These pathways are of potential therapeutic importance as targets for the prevention or treatment of neuropathogenesis.

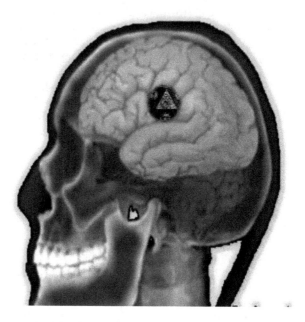

Figure 1. HIV virus can enter the CNS by altering the integrity of blood brain barrier.

4. Neuropathology of AIDS

HIV-1 is capable of causing a multi-system disorder including the CNS. HIV-1 enters the CNS at the early phase of infection, it persists and induces several motor and cognitive disorders leading to behavioural changes. Major clinical symptoms include impaired short term-memory, reduced mental concentration, weakness, slowness of hand and leg movement and depression accompanied by behavioural issues like personality disorders, lethargy and social withdrawal. These neurological and psychiatric symptoms caused by HIV-1 infection, constitute together as neuropathogenesis. A more subtle form of CNS dysfunction, known as minor cognitive motor disorder (MCMD), is also seen common in HIV patients. HAD cannot be controlled by HAART, HIV-1 infection becomes chronic and even rise in disease has been reported. The HIV-1 associated neuropathology is characterized by the infiltration of macrophages into the CNS, the formation of microglial nodules and multinucleated giant cells, astrocyte activation and damage; neuronal loss in ganglions and hippocampus, myelin damage, axonal damage and presence of HIV-1 in the CSF. MRI reports say that HIV infection is associated with progressive cortical atrophy which might be caused by neuronal loss and demyelination worsening in certain cognitive functions (Ghafouri et al., 2006).

5. HIV entry into the brain and initiation of HAD

HIV-1 infects cells having major HIV-1 receptors, CD4 and CD8, and several chemokine receptors which are known to be as HIV-1 co-receptors which help in the attachment of the virus to the cell and membrane fusion leading to viral entry. Infected CD4+ T cells and monocytes circulating in the blood are the potential source of CNS infection. HIV-1 infected cells can be either highly active producers or low/non producers of viruses. Both types of infections occur in the CNS. Studies of different astrocytes cell lines, demonstrated the presence of large quantities of Rev in the cytoplasm. Changes in cell environment, like the elevation in the level of cytokines such as TNF-α and IL-1β, might reactivate virus production (Ghafouri et al., 2006). During early infection, HIV enters the CNS (Bertin et al., 2012) and attacks cells macrophages and microglial cells (Foley et al., 2008). But along with this infection, periphery factors (non-CNS) are also important for initiating neurodegeneration and triggering dementia, which are like for example; increased number of circulating monocytes that express CD16 and CD69. The cells which get activated by viral entry, progressively adhere to the endothelium membrane of the brain microvasculature, and further transmigrate, triggering a spontaneous array of harmful processes which might finally lead to the loss of Blood Brain Barrier (BBB) integrity making it easy for virus to enter and replicate inside the brain. The BBB is crucial in HIV infection of the CNS. BBB is composed of specialized Human brain microvascular endothelial cells (HBMECs), which do not have any opening and are connected by intercellular junctions in an impermeable single layer. BBB plays a central role in neuropathogenesis as it serves as the channel through which free virus and infected immune cells enter the brain. The BBB loses its integrity and permeability due to progressive HIV infection and immune compromisation, which leads to easy entry of toxins, free virus, infected and activated monocytes into the brain. It has been reported that HIV-1 gp120 protein and also Tat protein are behind BBB disregulation. PKC signaling pathways and receptor-mediated Ca^{2+} release are the involved pathways resulting into cytotoxicity of the brain endothelial cells (Kanmogne et al., 2005) leading to downregulation and rupture of tight junction proteins (TJPs) of HBMECs, by the induction of proteasome by HIV-1. It has been studied that circulating virus or envelope proteins may also cause BBB dysfunction during primary infection. CNS infection of HIV is detected by viral RNA load in CSF (Woods et al., 2009; Morgan et al., 2011). Chemokines like monocyte chemoattractant protein (MCP)-1 control PBMCs relocation through BBB. Cellular migration engages adhesion molecules and differential regulation of inflammatory cytokines, leading to BBB disintegration and finally immune dysregulation by letting sufficient entry of infected or activated immune cells into the brain causing neuronal injury.

6. Types of CNS cells invaded by HIV-1

BBB is selectively permeable, made up of firmly concurrent brain microvascular endothelial cells, and its major role is to separate the CNS from the periphery. It manages the trafficking of cells and molecules across it into the brain parenchyma. For the purpose of brain entry, HIV-1 has to cross the BBB using several mechanisms which are still poorly understood and are unclear. Numerous *in vitro* experimentations have been done to understand the mechanisms of HIV-1 introduction into the CNS via BBB. It is reported that the severity of HIV-1 associated neuropathogenesis is dependent on amount of HIV DNA circulating in PBMCs (Shiramizu *et al.*, 2009). It is hypothesized that HIV-1 enters the CNS, in disguise as a commuter in cells trafficking till the brain (Verma *et al.*, 2010). CD4+ cells, like T cells and monocytes are infected by HIV-1, which circulate in blood and have the ability to cross the BBB and introduce the infection into CNS. Though presence of CD4 receptors in human brain microvascular endothelial cells is still a matter of debate whereas its presence is studied along with expression of HIV-1 co-receptors have also being reported on primary human brain's microvascular endothelial cells. Other proposed hypothesis for the entry of HIV-1 is the migration between/transcytosis of endothelial cells. All types of the CNS cells like astrocytes (Wang *et al.*, 2009), oligodendrocytes, neurons, macrophage and microglia, are easily infected by HIV-1 as they have receptors and co-receptors for HIV-1 entry, but only macrophage and microglia get infected most commonly which are the resident immunocompetent cells of the brain (Gendleman *et al.*, 1985). Expression of CCL2/MCP-1 in astrocytes is enhanced by nef via calmodulin dependent pathway. Consequently, increased CCL2/MCP-1 functions as a chemoattractant for monocytes, thereby facilitating entry of monocytes into the brain (Lehmann *et al.*, 2006). Peripheral macrophage population is necessary to be refilled, which is compensated by the migration of monocytes into the CNS, resulting in major drawback of facilitating the entry of intracellular virus. Microglia and monocyte-derived macrophages are the main culprits of HIV-1 CNS infection. Immunostaining experiments have shown HIV-1 infection in parenchymal microglia, but it is still unclear that whether the HIV-1 immunopositive microglia receives influx of infected cells from blood or directly results from prolonged infection in the CNS. *In-vitro* experiments demonstrate that HIV-1 replication takes place in primary microglia isolated from adults and infants leading to cytopathology. Microglial cells are the major targets as they express CD4/CCR5 major receptors/co-receptors which is a necessity for HIV-1 infection. On the other hand astrocytes express CXCR4 and other HIV-1 coreceptors like CCR5, but do not express CD4 receptors and are still reported to be infected by HIV-1 mechanisms to which are still unclear. Also *in vivo*, oligodendrocytes infection by HIV-1 remains unclear and less understood as they do not have CD4 receptors. Mostly there is absence of *in vivo* infection in neurons, however sometimes presence of HIV-1 DNA and proteins in neurons have been reported too, leading to need of further studies. Various pathways for the entry of virus into the brain have been studied like (i) direct entry, (ii) transcytosis, (iii) Trojan horse hypothesis for entry, which states that HIV enters the CNS via infected CD4 + AND T-cells which are capable of crossing BBB and they reach CNS and are also capable of transferring infection to other CNS cells too (Fig. 2).

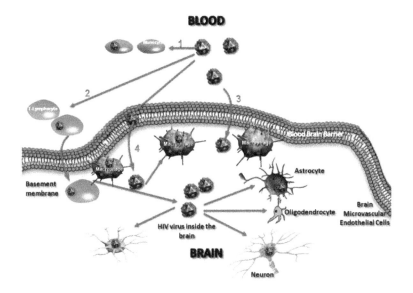

Figure 2. HIV-1 neuroinvasion. 1) "Trojan Horse hypothesis" for entry of HIV-1 into the brain via migration of infected monocytes which differentiate into perivascular macrophage. 2) The passage of infected CD4+ T cells into the brain. Other probable causes of CNS infection might be: 3) the direct entrance of the virus via tight junctions across the membrane and 4) entrance of HIV-1 by transcytosis phenomenon.

7. Crosstalk between the peripheral and CNS immunity

The way by which HIV-1-infected monocytes escape immune surveillance can be explained by "Trojan horse cell" model. The "support" needed for the viral entry is through CNS-produced chemokines like MCP-1 and IFN-γ-inducible peptide, CXCL10, whereas the "opposition" is through peripheral immune activation (Yadav et al., 2009). Upon entry in the brain, HIV-1-infected blood-borne macrophages secrete proinflammatory cytokines like tumor necrosis factor alpha (TNF-α), interleukin-1 beta (IL-1β), and viral proteins which affect neuronal function (Brabers and Nottet, 2006). Within the brain, astrocytes serve as principal regulators for neural homeostasis. They bring out a neurotoxic secretory response in macrophages, resulting to upregulation of certain acids and metabolites, chemokines, and cytokine secretions. They can also alter macrophage phenotype, which may help in neuroprotection. But on the contrary astrocytes can also influence autocrine and paracrine inflammatory cascades, which may lead to immune activation, increased viral infection, and allowance of cellular entry via BBB (Kraft-Terry *et al.*, 2010). Also CD16+ monocytes are linked to infection of the brain as they can be easily infected by the virus, they carry virus into the brain and help in viral dissemination and serve as viral reservoirs as they are apoptosis resistant. HIV proteins like nef require adaptive selection in brain for efficient replication in macrophages or when it is exposed to brain specific immune selection (Olivieri *et al.*, 2010). Neuropsychiatric disorders associated with HIV infection result in substantial morbidity and fatality. HIV injures the CNS and PNS, leading to neuropsychiatric disorders, which together constitute for neuroAIDS (McCombe *et al.*,2009), which includes neurocognitive disorders like HAD, minor neurocognitive disorder (HAND), mania, anxiety, depression, seizures, myelopathy and neuropathy, and also involves display of several symptoms like neurocognitive impairment, mood disorders, neuropathic pain, epilepsy, addiction, physical disability, loss of memory, mood swings etc (Fig.3).

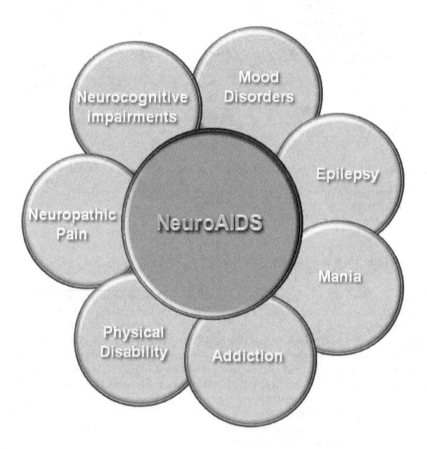

Figure 3. Associated disorders and symptoms which are commonly seen in patients suffering from neuroAIDS.

8. Forms of dementia

One form of dementia is Alzheimer's disease caused by amyloid pathology, during which peptides of amyloid-β generate and clump together into plaques which release toxic fragments of amyloid-β leading to neuropathogenesis. Another form of dementia is caused by vascular pathology in which blood vessels leak and hence deprives small areas of the brain of blood and oxygen, which damage brain tissue resulting in cognitive defects. Both forms exist equally, even though Alzheimer pathology is more common, but it coexists with vascular pathology. (Abott *et al.*, 2011).

TYPES OF DEMENTIA			
Dementia type	Symptoms	Neuropathological findings	Percentage of total dementia cases
Alzheimer's	Weakened memory power, leading to confusion, disinterest depression and bad judgement skills.	Formation of amyloid plaques and also neurofibrillary tangles.	50–80%
Vascular dementia	Memory is weakened, but not as intense as in the case of Alzheimer's patients.	Causing microstrokes due to reduced blood flow to brain	20–30%
Frontotemporal dementia	Personality disorders, mood swings and difficulty in understanding different languages.	Damage limited to frontal and temporal lobes	5–10%
Dementia with Lewy bodies	Weakened memory power, leading to confusion, disinterest depression and bad judgement skills, hallucinations and tremors.	Cortical Lewy bodies (of the protein a-synuclein) inside neurons.	<5%

Table 1. Displaying the types of dementia and their prevalance. (Source: Abbott A. Dementia: a problem for our age. *Nature.* 2011; 475(7355): S2-4)

9. Knowing dementia and its diagnosis

Dementia is considered as loss of memory and other cognitive abilities which reduces the lifespan of patients. Dementia is often associated with physical, mental and financial burden. 37% of the dementic population in developing countries have vulnerable living environment and they require specialised care. Diagnosis of dementia involves investigations for decline in memory and disturbance in several cognitive abilities like coherent speech, understanding spoken or written language, recognizing objects, executing motor activities, sensory function, thinking abstractly, making sound judgments, planning and carrying out complex tasks. Dementia reduces the lifespan of affected people. In the developed countries life span after dementia diagnosis can be expected to be ~7 years, but in low and middle income countries survival may be shorter. Dementia symptoms and linked issues can be understood in three stages of early stage (1-2 years) which is often overlooked because the onset of dementia is gradual, making it difficult to predict when it begins, leading to problems in talking, memory loss. Secondly, the middle stage (2-5 years) which makes patients life more difficult and restricted, giving them difficulty in day-to-day living and forgetting recent events and people's names, etc. Thirdly, the late stage (>5 years) leading to total dependence and inactivity, serious memory disturbances difficulty in physical works like walking, eating, incapability of communicating, not recognizing familiar objects, displaying inappropriate behavior in public etc.

HIV associated dementia, referred as the syndrome of cognitive and motor dysfunction resulting in progressive neurodegeneration observed after infection with human HIV-1, also known as HIV encephalopathy (HIV-E) and AIDS dementia complex (ADC) (Kaul et al., 2001). In the last stage of HIV, HAD a severe neurological complication affects 15–20% of the patients (Van de Bovenkamp et al., 2002). The relationship between spreading of HIV in brain tissue and pathology has not been thoroughly assessed in HAART era (Lamers et al., 2010). Inspite of preventing former end stage complications of AIDS by HAART however, with increased survival times, the prevalence of minor HIV-1 associated cognitive impairment appears to be rising among AIDS patients. Further, HIV-1 associated dementia (HAD) is still prevalent in treated patients as well as attenuated forms of HAD and CNS opportunistic disorders (Ghafouri et al., 2006). Infected macrophages with HIV have an ability to cross BBB infect inhabitant brain macrophages initiating the development of HAD. Cytokines are released from infected resident brain macrophages which further attract more macrophages to sites of infection and a series of self-inflammatory process emerges (Williams et al., 2002). Studies have suggested that the process of entering in the CNS causing HAD mostly depends on the HIV variants as some HIV variants have capability of entering in the CNS and develops HAD but in contrast other variants don't have capability to develop HAD even after entering in the CNS (Fischer-Smith et al., 2008; Fischer-Smith et al., 2005).

10. Underlying mechanisms and issues

Some studies suggest that neurological involvement of infected patients occurs at different frequencies, depending on the HIV subtype involved in the infection (Liner 2nd et al., 2007). HIV-1 Subtype D has more prominent chance for developing dementia (89%) than subtype A (24%) in the patients localized in a region of Uganda, Africa suggesting genetic determinants exist within HIV that influence the ability of the virus to replicate in the central nervous system. HIV-1 proteins have been shown to be released from HIV infected cell and/ or they have found to be present in the extracellular milieu in the HIV-1-

infected brain. In vitro, neurotoxic and/or neuromodulatory effects have been shown by HIV proteins: nef, env, tat, rev, vpr and vpu that might play a role in the development of HIV-1-associated dementia in vivo (Sactor *et al.*, 2009).

11. Fight against dementia

Dementia is engulfing bigger proportion of HIV patients and is expected to worsen more. It is expected that a significant proportion of dementia is driven by amyloid-β. But so far none of the amyloid-based strategies has been successful, but still drug developers are strategising on the concept which can combat against it. More reliable biomarkers are being developed potentially making it possible to carry out trials on patients before symptoms. Some scientists are also wondering to target vascular pathology as well, which is equally responsible for causing dementia. So cholesterol level lowering drugs and blood pressure reducing drugs are also given long term to patients, who are at higher risk of heart attack which may also help protect from dementias as well (Abott *et al.*, 2011). There are several extracellular and intra-cellular signalling pathways, which when activated lead to macrophage or microglial activation, and induction in neurons and astrocytes. These pathways may act as a potential therapeutic importance as drug targets against neuropathogenesis. NeuroAIDS is challenge to patients, their families, society and our country, thus development of preclinical models appropriate for new compounds testing with neurotrophic and neuroprotective potential is necessary (Crews *et al.*, 2008; Williams *et al.*, 2008).

12. Therapeutic developments

The biggest issue which comes in front of drug developers is the incapability of the drugs to cross the BBB, which leads to low bioavailability of the drugs into the CNS. HIV-1 protease inhibitors are totally incapable in entering the CNS, while other HIV-1 therapies such as zidovudine (AZT) are reported to have efficient BBB penetration. Recently, a broad range of nanomedicines are being developed to improve drug delivery across BBB, development of nanoparticulate– antiretroviral therapy (nanoART), against CNS disorders as the structure of the BBB, efflux pumps and the expression of metabolic enzymes make it difficult for the regular drug to reach brain. Nanoformulations can evade the BBB and can boost CNS-directed drug delivery (Fig. 4) (Saxena *et al.*, 2012; Nowacek *et al.*, 2010; Nowacek *et al.*, 2009). Efforts are been done in finding long-lasting injectable antiretrovirals to avoid the challenges of therapy adherence (Baert *et al.*, 2009). To specifically target the CNS, NPs are synthesized with various combinations of ART therapies to be taken up by monocytes and carried into the CNS for release at sites of HIV-1 infection, for example Indinavir nanoART and p24 loaded and coated NP, which are providing new avenues for treating or even preventing the spread of HIV-1 in the brain. Adjunctive therapeutics ART is engaged in making combinatory drugs against virus mutation. Efforts are being made to improve penetrability of ART across the BBB, but importance of considering drug toxicity and elicited cellular response for various ART regiments is always a necessity. Adjunctive therapy like platelet-activating factor (PAF) antagonist, PMS-601, are demonstrated to reduce HAND symptoms and even combination of ART and PAF antagonists, are also studied to have role in reducing neurodegeneration. All of these are also being developed as therapies for neurodegenerative disorders which may prove to be a boon in the combat against NeuroAIDS. Need of the hour is to device an exact combination of CNS-penetrating nanoART and adjunctive therapies, which might be able to help us against neurocognitive symptoms (Kraft-Terry *et al.*, 2010).

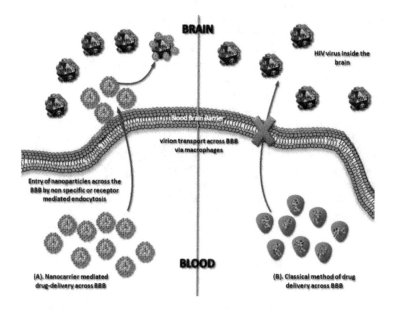

Figure 4. Comparative display of nanocarrier mediated method of drug delivery (A) versus the classical method of drug delivery across the Blood Brain Barrier (BBB), which is less efficient than the former in the process of drug delivery.

13. Future implications and need of the hour

Since dementia is quite prevalent in HIV patients, in developed countries and has also been reported to extend its grip towards developing countries as well due to increase in patient survival rates and life expectancy due to HAART treatment and increased living standards. Low prevalence of HAD in underdeveloped and developing countries have been attributed to under diagnosis, short life expectancy and short survival following HIV infection associated with opportunistic infections and also low prevalence of HIV related neuroinfections and pathology is not available due to inadequate medical facilities, social stigma and ignorance that lead to under diagnosis (Vivithanaporn *et al.*, 2010). So a need of collaboratory studies is there which can be used, for learning the cause, prevalence and diagnosis of neuropathogenesis. A synchronised effort is needed by researchers, drug makers, physicians, policy makers, government bodies nationally as well as globally. A proper and deep understanding about the entry of the virus into the CNS and the various mechanisms it employs to undertake the host machinery would be of great help in understanding the issue and combating against the virus.

Author details

Shailendra K. Saxena[1], Sneham Tiwari[1] and Madhavan P.N. Nair[2]

1 Centre for Cellular and Molecular Biology (CCMB-CSIR), Hyderabad, India

2 College of Medicine, Florida International University, Miami, USA

References

[1] Abbott, A. (2011). Dementia: a problem for our age." *Nature*. 475(7355): S, 2-4.

[2] Baert, L, Klooster, t, Dries, G, François, W, Wouters, M, Basstanie, A, Iterbeke, E, Stappers, K, Stevens, F, Schueller, P, Van Remoortere, L, Kraus, P, Wigerinck, G, & Rosier, P. J. ((2009). Development of a long-acting injectable formulation with nano-particles of rilpivirine (TMC278) for HIV treatment." *Eur J Pharm Biopharm*. 72(3), 502-508.

[3] Bertin, J, Barat, C, Méthot, S, & Tremblay, M. J. (2012). Interactions between prosta-glandins, leukotrienes and HIV-1: possible implications for the central nervous sys-tem." *Retrovirology*. 9:4.

[4] Brabers, N. A, & Nottet, H. S. (2006). Role of the pro-inflammatory cytokines TNF-alpha and IL-1beta in HIV-associated dementia." *Eur J Clin Invest*. , 36(7), 447-458.

[5] Crews, L, Lentz, M. R, Gonzalez, R. G, Fox, H. S, & Masliah, E. (2008). Neuronal in-jury in simian immunodeficiency virus and other animal models of neuroAIDS." *J Neurovirol*. , 14(4), 327-339.

[6] Dean, D, & Berger, J. R. (2012). Neuro-AIDS in the developing world." *Neurology*. , 78(7), 499-500.

[7] Ferris, M. J, Mactutus, C. F, & Booze, R. M. (2008). Neurotoxic profiles of HIV, psy-chostimulant drugs of abuse, and their concerted effect on the brain: current status of dopamine system vulnerability in NeuroAIDS." *Neurosci Biobehav Rev*. , 32(5), 883-909.

[8] Fischer-smith, T, & Rappaport, J. (2005). Evolving paradigms in the pathogenesis of HIV-1-associated dementia." *Expert Rev Mol Med*. , 7(27), 1-26.

[9] Fischer-smith, T, Bell, C, Croul, S, Lewis, M, & Rappaport, J. (2008). Monocyte/ macrophage trafficking in acquired immunodeficiency syndrome encephalitis: lessons from human and nonhuman primate studies." *J Neurovirol.* , 14(4), 318-326.

[10] Foley, J, Ettenhofer, M, Wright, M, & Hinkin, C. H. (2008). Emerging issues in the neuropsychology of HIV infection." *Curr HIV/AIDS Rep.* , 5(4), 204-211.

[11] Gandhi, N, Saiyed, Z. M, Napuri, J, Samikkannu, T, Reddy, P. V, Agudelo, M, Khatavkar, P, Saxena, S. K, & Nair, M. P. (2010). Interactive role of human immunodeficiency virus type 1 (HIV-1) clade-specific Tat protein and cocaine in blood-brain barrier dysfunction: implications for HIV-1-associated neurocognitive disorder." *J Neurovirol.* , 16(4), 294-305.

[12] Gendelman, H. E, Narayan, O, Molineaux, S, Clements, J. E, & Ghotbi, Z. (1985). Slow, persistent replication of lentiviruses: role of tissue macrophages and macrophage precursors in bone marrow." *Proc Natl Acad Sci U S A.* , 82(20), 7086-7090.

[13] Ghafouri, M, Amini, S, Khalili, K, & Sawaya, B. E. (2006). HIV-1 associated dementia: symptoms and causes." *Retrovirology.* 19;3: 28.

[14] Kanmogne, G. D, Primeaux, C, & Grammas, P. (2005). HIV-1 gp120 proteins alter tight junction protein expression and brain endothelial cell permeability: implications for the pathogenesis of HIV-associated dementia." *J Neuropathol Exp Neurol.* , 64(6), 498-505.

[15] Kaul, M, Garden, G. A, & Lipton, S. A. (2001). Pathways to neuronal injury and apoptosis in HIV-associated dementia." *Nature.* , 410(6831), 988-994.

[16] Kilareski, E. M, Shah, S, Nonnemacher, M. R, & Wigdahl, B. (2009). Regulation of HIV-1 transcription in cells of the monocyte-macrophage lineage." *Retrovirology.* 6:118.

[17] Kraft-terry, S. D, Stothert, A. R, Buch, S, & Gendelman, H. E. (2010). HIV-1 neuroimmunity in the era of antiretroviral therapy." Neurobiol Dis. , 37(3), 542-548.

[18] Lamers, S. L, Poon, A. F, & Mcgrath, M. S. (2011). HIV-1 nef protein structures associated with brain infection and dementia pathogenesis." *PLoS One.* 6(2): e16659.

[19] Lamers, S. L, Salemi, M, Galligan, D. C, Morris, A, Gray, R, Fogel, G, Zhao, L, & Mcgrath, M. S. (2010). Human immunodeficiency virus-1 evolutionary patterns associated with pathogenic processes in the brain." *J Neurovirol.* , 16(3), 230-241.

[20] Lehmann, M. H, Masanetz, S, Kramer, S, & Erfle, V. (2006). HIV-1 Nef upregulates CCL2/MCP-1 expression in astrocytes in a myristoylation- and calmodulin-dependent manner." *J Cell Sci.* 119(Pt 21): 4520-4530.

[21] Liner, K. J. nd, Hall, C.D. and Robertson, K.R. ((2007). Impact of human immunodeficiency virus (HIV) subtypes on HIV-associated neurological disease." *J Neurovirol.* , 13(4), 291-304.

[22] Mccombe, J. A, Noorbakhsh, F, Buchholz, C, Trew, M, & Power, C. (2009). Neuro-AIDS: a watershed for mental health and nervous system disorders." *J Psychiatry Neurosci.* , 34(2), 83-85.

[23] Morgan, E. E, Woods, S. P, Delano-wood, L, & Bondi, M. W. Grant I; HIV Neurobehavioral Research Program (HNRP) Group. ((2011). Intraindividual variability in HIV infection: evidence for greater neurocognitive dispersion in older HIV seropositive adults." *Neuropsychology.* , 25(5), 645-654.

[24] Nowacek, A, & Gendelman, H. E. (2009). NanoART, neuroAIDS and CNS drug delivery." *Nanomedicine* (Lond). , 4(5), 557-574.

[25] Nowacek, A. S, Mcmillan, J, Miller, R, Anderson, A, Rabinow, B, & Gendelman, H. E. (2010). Nanoformulated antiretroviral drug combinations extend drug release and antiretroviral responses in HIV-1-infected macrophages: implications for neuroAIDS therapeutics." *J Neuroimmune Pharmacol.* Epub, 5(4), 592-601.

[26] Olivieri, K. C, Agopian, K. A, Mukerji, J, & Gabuzda, D. (2010). Evidence for adaptive evolution at the divergence between lymphoid and brain HIV-1 nef genes." *AIDS Res Hum Retroviruses.* , 26(4), 495-500.

[27] Prince, M, Acosta, D, Ferri, C. P, Guerra, M, & Huang, Y. Llibre Rodriguez, J.J.,Salas, A., Sosa, A.L., Williams, J.D., Dewey, M.E., Acosta, I., Jotheeswaran, A.T. and Liu, Z. ((2012). Dementia incidence and mortality in middle-income countries, and associations with indicators of cognitive reserve: a 10/66 Dementia Research Group population-based cohort study." *Lancet.* 380(9836), 50-58.

[28] Prince, M, Brodaty, H, Uwakwe, R, Acosta, D, Ferri, C. P, Guerra, M, Huang, Y, & Jacob, K. S. Llibre Rodriguez, J.J., Salas, A., Sosa, A.L., Williams, J.D., Jotheeswaran, A.T. and Liu, Z. ((2012). Strain and its correlates among carers of people with dementia in low-income and middle-income countries. A 10/66 Dementia Research Group population-based survey." *Int J Geriatr Psychiatry.* , 27(7), 670-82.

[29] Reddy, P. V, Pilakka-kanthikee, S, Saxena, S. K, Saiyed, Z, & Nair, M. P. (2012). Interactive Effects of Morphine on HIV Infection: Role in HIV-Associated Neurocognitive Disorder." *AIDS Res Treat.* 2012: 953678.

[30] Sacktor, N, Nakasujja, N, Robertson, K, & Clifford, D. B. (2007). HIV-associated cognitive impairment in sub-Saharan Africa--the potential effect of clade diversity." *Nat Clin Pract Neurol.* , 3(8), 436-443.

[31] Sacktor, N, Nakasujja, N, Skolasky, R. L, Rezapour, M, Robertson, K, Musisi, S, & Quinn, T. C. (2009). HIV subtype D is associated with dementia, compared with subtype A, in immunosuppressed individuals at risk of cognitive impairment in Kampala, Uganda." *Clin Infect Dis.* , 49(5), 780-786.

[32] Saiyed, Z. M, Gandhi, N, Agudelo, M, Napuri, J, Samikkannu, T, Reddy, P. V, Khatavkar, P, Yndart, A, Saxena, S. K, & Nair, M. P. (2011). HIV-1 Tat upregulates ex-

pression of histone deacetylase-2 (HDAC2) in human neurons: implication for HIV-associated neurocognitive disorder (HAND)." *Neurochem Int.* , 58(6), 656-64.

[33] Samikkannu, T, Rao, K. V, Gandhi, N, Saxena, S. K, & Nair, M. P. (2010). Human immunodeficiency virus type 1 clade B and C Tat differentially induce indoleamine 2,3-dioxygenase and serotonin in immature dendritic cells: Implications for neuroAIDS." *J Neurovirol.* , 16(4), 255-263.

[34] Saxena, S. K, Gupta, A, Bhagyashree, K, Saxena, R, Arora, N, Banerjee, A. K, Tripathi, A. K, Chandrasekar, M. J, Gandhi, N, & Nair, M. P. (2012). Targeting strategies for Human immunodeficiency virus: a combinatorial approach." *Mini Rev Med Chem.* , 12(3), 236-254.

[35] Saxena, S. K, Shrivastava, G, Tiwari, S, & Nair, M. P. N. (2012). HIV-1 Nef: hacker of the host cell." *Future Virol.* 7(2), 117-120

[36] Saxena, S. K, Shrivastava, G, Tiwari, S, Swamy, M. A, & Nair, M. P. (2012). Modulation of HIV pathogenesis and T-cell signaling by HIV-1 Nef." *Future Virol.* , 7(6), 609-620.

[37] Saxena, S. K, Tiwari, S, & Nair, M. P. (2012). Nanotherapeutics: emerging competent technology in neuroAIDS and CNS drug delivery." *Nanomedicine (Lond).* , 7(7), 941-944.

[38] Saxena, S. K, Tiwari, S, & Nair, M. P. (2012). A global perspective on HIV/AIDS." *Science.* 337(6096): 798.

[39] Shankar, S. K, Mahadevan, A, Satishchandra, P, Kumar, R. U, Yasha, T. C, Santosh, V, Chandramuki, A, Ravi, V, & Nath, A. (2005). Neuropathology of HIV/AIDS with an overview of the Indian scene." *Indian J Med Res.* 121(4), 468-488.

[40] Shiramizu, B, Williams, A. E, Shikuma, C, & Valcour, V. (2009). Amount of HIV DNA in peripheral blood mononuclear cells is proportional to the severity of HIV-1-associated neurocognitive disorders." *J Neuropsychiatry Clin Neurosci.* , 21(1), 68-74.

[41] Singh, R, Kaur, M, & Arora, D. (2011). Neurological complications in late-stage hospitalized patients with HIV disease." *Ann Indian Acad Neurol.* , 14(3), 172-177.

[42] Sundaravaradan, V, Saxena, S. K, Ramakrishnan, R, Yedavalli, V. R, Harris, D. T, & Ahmad, N. (2006). Differential HIV-1 replication in neonatal and adult blood mononuclear cells is influenced at the level of HIV-1 gene expression." *Proc Natl Acad Sci U S A.* , 103(31), 11701-11706.

[43] Van de BovenkampM., Nottet, H.S. and Pereira, C.F. ((2002). Interactions of human immunodeficiency virus-1 proteins with neurons: possible role in the development of human immunodeficiency virus-1-associated dementia." *Eur J Clin Invest.* , 32(8), 619-627.

[44] Verma, A. S, Singh, U. P, Dwivedi, P. D, & Singh, A. (2010). Contribution of CNS cells in NeuroAIDS." *J Pharm Bioallied Sci.* , 2(4), 300-306.

[45] Vivithanaporn, P, Heo, G, Gamble, J, Krentz, H. B, Hoke, A, Gill, M. J, & Power, C. (2010). Neurologic disease burden in treated HIV/AIDS predicts survival: a population-based study." *Neurology.* , 75(13), 1150-1158.

[46] Wang, T, Gong, N, Liu, J, Kadiu, I, Kraft-terry, S. D, Schlautman, J. D, Ciborowski, P, Volsky, D. J, & Gendelman, H. E. (2008). HIV-1-infected astrocytes and the microglial proteome." *J Neuroimmune Pharmacol.* , 3(3), 173-186.

[47] Williams, K. C, & Hickey, W. F. (2002). Central nervous system damage, monocytes and macrophages, and neurological disorders in AIDS." *Annu Rev Neurosci.* , 25, 537-562.

[48] Williams, R, Bokhari, S, Silverstein, P, Pinson, D, Kumar, A, & Buch, S. (2008). Non-human primate models of NeuroAIDS." *J Neurovirol.* 14(4), 292-300.

[49] Woods, S. P, Moore, D. J, Weber, E, & Grant, I. (2009). Cognitive neuropsychology of HIV-associated neurocognitive disorders." *Neuropsychol Rev.* , 19(2), 152-168.

[50] Yadav, A, & Collman, R. G. (2009). CNS inflammation and macrophage/microglial biology associated with HIV-1 infection." *J Neuroimmune Pharmacol.* , 4(4), 430-447.

Chapter 7

Neurological Manifestations of HIV-1 Infection and Markers for HIV Progression

Rehana Basri and Wan Mohamad Wan Majdiah

Additional information is available at the end of the chapter

1. Introduction

Human immunodeficiency virus, or HIV, is the virus that causes acquired immune deficiency syndrome (AIDS). The acquired immunodeficiency syndrome (AIDS) was first described in 1981 in USA. In 1983, human immunodeficiency virus type-1 (HIV-1) was isolated, and in the following year it was demonstrated clearly that it was the causative agent of AIDS. The disease is a major health problem in many parts of the world. The high prevalence and striking diversity of neurological disorders complicating AIDS were recognized in 1983 (Snider et al., 1983). AIDS was associated with distinct neurological syndromes, such as dementia, myelopathy and painful neuropathy that appeared to result from the HIV itself. Over the last 30 years, there has been increasing recognition of the role that auto antibodies play in neurological disorders. During the past decade, AIDS has become a global health problem with 182,000 000 cases reported from 152 countries. It is estimated that nearly five to ten million people are infected worldwide with HIV-1. With a mean incubation period from time of infection to the development of AIDS of eight to 10 years, it is projected that nearly all HIV-1-infected individual will develop AIDS within the next 15 years (Quinn, 1990). It has become increasingly evident that the vast majority of HIV-1 infected people will eventually develop AIDS or an AIDS-related condition (De Wolf and Lange, 1991) with a median time of progression to AIDS of 7-10 years from infection in adults (Lui et al., 1988; Bacchetti and Moss, 1989) and shorter periods in infants and elderly patients (Medley et al., 1987; Auger et al., 1988; Lagakos & DeGruttola, 1989). In the United States alone, 104, 210 cases of AIDS and more than 61,000 deaths have been reported. Sexual, parenteral as well as perinatal transmission routes have remained the major modes of transmission, although the proportion of cases within each risk behaviour category has changed. Recently, there has been a dramatic increase in the proportion of AIDS patients who have acknowledged as IV drug user or have heterosexual contact with other individuals at high risk for HIV infection (Quinn, 1990).

In Sub-Saharan Africa, 22.5 million people living with HIV (68% of the global infections) and 1.6 million AIDS death in 2007 (76% of the AIDS deaths worldwide). In recent years, global efforts have increased substantially. The most encouraging improvements have been in Sub-Saharan Africa where the number of people being treated with anti-retrovirals has increased tenfold from 2003 to 2006 (Peters et al., 2008). The decline of HIV infection in some regions was partially offset by a rise in new infections in other parts of the globe, particularly in Asia and Eastern Europe (Delpech & Gahagan, 2009). It was estimated that over 5 million people in South Asia living with HIV/AIDS. Almost 90% of those infected live in India. Other countries in the region such as Bangladesh, Pakistan and Nepal have a low HIV prevalence in general population (Abeysena & De Silva, 2005).

2. Back ground of immune defence mechanisms

Humoral immunity and complement system: immunity that is mediated by secreted antibodies produced in the cells of the B lymphocyte. Cell mediated immunity : is an immune response that does not involve antibodies but rather involves the activation of macrophages, natural (NK), antigen-specific cytotoxic T-lymphocytes.

2.1. Causes of immunosuppression primary: Antibody deficiency, combined antibody

Antibody deficiency, combined antibody and cellular deficiency, Complement deficiency. Acquired: Extremes of age, Diabetes, Chronic alcoholism, HIV infection, Connective tissue diseases, Organ failure (renal, hepatic), Malignancy, Iatrogenic (chemotherapy, radiotherapy, Transplantation). HIV is a retrovirus that primarily infects vital organs of the human immune system such as CD4+ T cells (a subset of T cells), macrophages and dendritic cells. It directly and indirectly destroys CD4+ T cells (Alimonti et al 2003).

2.2. Cells affected

The virus entering through which ever route and acts primarily on the following cells: Lymphoreticular system: CD_4+ T-Helper cells, Macrophages, Monocytes, B-lymphocytes, Certain endothelial cells and Central nervous system: Microglia, Astrocytes, Oligodendrocytes, and Neurones.

2.3. Relation of CD4 T cell count

Neurologic Complications increase with decline in CD_4 T cell count. CD_4 T cell count > 500/µl – Early stage – Demyelinating Neuropathies, CD_4 T cell count 200 to 500 – Mid stage – Dementia - VZV radiculities and CD_4 T cell count <200 –advance stage → Dementia, Myelopathy, Painful-neuropathy.

2.4. Immune deficiency & clinical disease

Clinical manifestations, Susceptibility to infections, Lymphoreticular malignancies, autoimmune disease.

3. Neurological menifestations of HIV-1 infections

HIV is neuroinvasive, it does not directly infect neurons. The major brain reservoirs for HIV infection and replication are microglia and macrophages. Astrocytes can be infected but are not a site of active HIV replication. HIV-associated neurologic complications are indirect effects of viral neurotoxins (viral proteins gp120 and tat) and neurotoxins released by infected or activated microglia, macrophages and astrocytes. Neurologic manifestations occur over the entire spectrum of HIV disease. Fifty to 70% of patients experienced acute clinical syndrome 1 to 6 wks after infection, Neuro Manifestations occur in 10% involves Multiple Parts of nervous system. Some Monophonic illness Meningitis, Meningioencephalitis, Seizures, Myelopathy, Cranial and Peripheral Neuropathy linked to primary HIV and recover within 1 week. Neurological opportunistic infections and malignancies predominated in early reports, but it became also clear that AIDS was associated with distinct neurological syndromes, such as Acute/subacute diffuse encephalopathy Progressive dementia, Focal mass lesions, Acute stroke like presentation, Meningitis, Multiple cranial neuropathies and Acute/subacute myelopathy.

3.1. HIV encephalopathy

(AIDS Dementia Complex or HIV associated Dementia) is a late complication of HIV infection and progresses slowly over months seen in pts with CD_{4T} cell Count >350cells/μl. Dementia is a major feature but aphasia, apraxia and afnofia uncommon, motor abnormality like unsteady gait, poor balance, tremor and in late stage develop apathy & lack of initiative – leads to vegetative state mania (table 1). Neuro imaging: MRI & CT demonstrate cerebral atrophy, Basal ganglia calcification in children. CSF: MonoNucleatz cells increase, Protein increase, RNA can be detected and HIV can be cultured. Infective: CMV ventriculoencephalitis, Varicella encephalitis, Herpes encephalitis, Toxoplasma encephalitis (rare).

Table 1. Clinical staging of HIV Encephalopathy

Treatment:

Combination anti retro viral therapy is beneficial and rapid improvement in cognitive function.

3.2. HIV-associated dementia

The major direct effect of HIV infection on the immune system is the profound and progressive loss of CD4 lymphocytes. This leads to impaired cellular immunity, and a dysregulation of macrophages, with the overproduction of a variety of proinflammatory cytokines and chemokines (Griffin, 1997). HIV can enter the nervous system early after infection, but productive infection is rarely detectable before immunosuppression has developed. Based upon phylogenetic analysis of HIV gp160, the route of central nervous system (CNS) infection appears to primarily involve infected monocytes (Liu et al., 2000) as well as free viral particles and HIV proteins crossing a disrupted blood–brain barrier. The presentation of HIV-D includes cognitive, behavioral, and motor dysfunction, and suggests a predominant subcortical involvement (Navia et al., 1986). In the early stages, memory loss, mental slowing, reading and comprehension difficulties, and apathy are frequent com plaints (Fig. 1) (Mc Arthur et al., 2003).

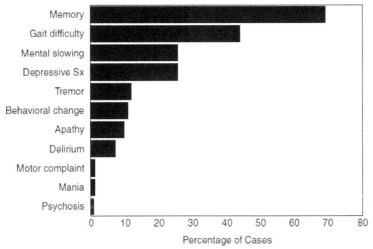

Figure 1. Frequency of symptoms in HIV dementia among 300 subjects personally examined at JHU HIV Neurology program (McArthur et al., 2003).

The cognitive deficits of HIV- D are characterized primarily by (1) memory loss that is selective for impaired retrieval; (2) impaired ability to manipulate acquired knowledge; (3) personality changes including apathy, inertia, and irritability; and (4) general slowing of all thought processes. Gait disturbance and impairment of fine manual dexterity are common early manifestations. Examination findings include impaired rapid movements of eyes and limbs, diffuse hyperreflexia, frontal release signs, and sometimes Parkinsonism (Mirsattari et al., 1998). A recent study suggests that antiretroviral drug combinations with drugs that have better CSF penetration are associated with greater CSF viral load suppression and may be associated with greater improvement in neuropsychological test deficits compared to antiretroviral drug combinations with drugs that have poor CSF penetration (Letendre et al., 2004). Antiretroviral drugs with the highest CSF:plasma ratios or with profound effects on viral replication in the periphery with a resulting decrease in virus entry into the CNS (e.g., zidovudine, stavudine, abacavir, nevirapine, efavirenz, and indinavir) are likely to be the most efficacious for the treatment of HIV-D. Affective: Apathy (depression-like features), Irritability, Mania, new onset psychosis. Behavioral: Psychomotor retardation (slowed speech or response time), Personality changes, Social withdrawal. Cognitive: Lack of visuospatial memory (misplacing things), Lack of vasomotor coordination, Difficulty with complex sequencing (difficulty in performing previously learned complex tasks), Impaired concentration and attention-Impaired verbal memory (word-finding ability), Mental slowing. Motor: Unsteady gait, loss of balance, Leg weakness, dropping things, Tremors, poor handwriting and decline in fine motor skills.

3.3. HIV associated neuropathy

Symptomatic neuropathies occur in approximately 10% to 15%. Pathologic evidence of peripheral nerve involvement is present in virtually all end-stage AIDS patients. The most common complaints are numbness, parethesias and painful dysestesias. Zanetti et al., (2004) reported mild distal dysestesia that neither interfered with the activities of daily living nor required specific therapy. The main neurological sign was distal symmetric sensory alteration (in 97.1% of the patients) in the four limbs but mainly in the feet. The etiology and pathogenesis of peripheral neuropathy associated with HIV infection is uncertain. It can be caused by the direct or indirect action of HIV and antibody production, or secondary to infections (CMV, MAC), toxic effects of certain drugs (isoniazid, vincristine, d4T, ddi, ddC), or nutritional deficiencies (vitamin B12) (Rizzuto et al., 1995; Dalakas et al., 1988; Figg, 1991; Browne et al., 1993; Pike, 1993; Abrams et al., 1994; Kieburtz et al., 1991; Norton et al., 1996; Gill et al., 1990; Simpson et al.,1995). Almost all patients with HIV that had diagnosis of peripheral neuropathy were taking drugs probably neurotoxic (ddi, d4t,ddC isoniazid) (Zanetti et al., 2004) to determine the effect of 5 weeks of individualized acupuncture treatment, delivered in a group setting, on pain and symptoms of peripheral neuropathy associated with HIV infection. In addition, the acupuncture regimen reduced pain/aching/burning and pins/needles/numbness in the upper and lower limbs (Phillips et al., 2004).

3.4. HIV related to myelopathy with polyradiculopathy

The most common cause of spinal cord disease in AIDS patients is AIDS-associated myelopathy, with a reported prevalence of 20% to 55% in different series (Gray et al., 1990; Henin et al., 1992; Petito et al., 1985; Goldstick, 1985; Dal et al., 1994; Artigas et al., 1990). Clinical symptoms and signs of myelopathy included spastic paraparesis, gait disturbance, urinary problems, and impotence in males, hyperreflexia, and a variable degree of sensory loss. A clinical rating of the severity of the myelopathy was established by a neurologist blinded to the MR findings. The myelopathy was rated as mild, moderate, or severe: mild if there were only subjective complaints of leg stiffness, heaviness, cramps, or subjective bladder dysfunction (not incontinence), together with objective findings of increased tone, hyperreflexia, or extensor plantar responses; moderate if there was objectively demonstrable weakness of the lower extremities or incontinence; and severe if the patient was not independently ambulatory. The MR findings of the spinal cord were subsequently correlated with the clinical rating of the severity of the myelopathy. June et al, 1999, reported spinal cord MR features were abnormal in 18 (86%) of the 21 patients (table 2). The most common finding was spinal cord atrophy, seen in 15 patients (71%) (Fig 2).

MR Findings in the Spinal Cord	No. of Patients	Clinical Rating of Severity of Myelopathy, No. (%)		
		Mild	Moderate	Severe
Normal MR findings	3	2 (66.7)	0	1 (33.3)
Cord atrophy	15	3 (20.0)	9 (60.0)	3 (20.0)
Intrinsic cord signal abnormality	6	1 (16.7)	2 (33.3)	3 (50.0)
Atrophy plus cord signal abnormality	3	1 (33.3)	0	2 (66.7)

Table 2. American Journal of Neuroradiology 20:1412-1416 (9 1999)

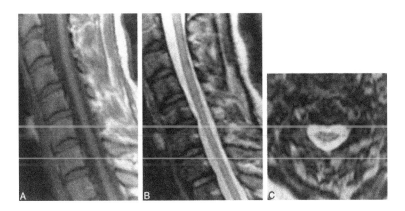

Figure 2. American Journal of Neuroradiology 20:1412-1416 (9 1999)

AIDS-associated myelopathy is characterized pathologically by discrete or coalescent intramyelin and periaxonal vacuolation, with cellular debris and lipid-laden macrophages, in the white matter of the spinal cord. The axons are usually intact, but in severe vacuolization, they may become disrupted. It typically involves the lateral and posterior columns of the cervical and thoracic cord (Henin et al., 1992; Petito et al., 1985; Dal et al., 1994; Tan et al., 1995). The effect of HAART on improving the symptoms or slowing the progression of HIV-associated myelopathy is not known. A pilot study using high doses of oral L-methionine led to improvement in clinical and electrophysiologic features of the disease in an open-label clinical trial (Dorfman et al., 1997). Uncontrolled clinical experience no benefit from corticosteroids and intravenous immunoglobulin (IVIG).

3.5. HIV-Associated Neuromuscular Weakness Syndrome (HANWS)

Toxic events secondary to use of HAART can be observed globally. Recently, Simpson et al. 2004, reported a heterogeneous syndrome termed the HIV-associated neuromuscular weakness syndrome (HANWS) which seems to be related to hyperlactatemia and stavudine and/or didanosine exposure. Rapidly ascending neuromuscular weakness syndrome," associated with lactic acidosis syndrome in HIV-infected patients. Majority dramatic motor weakness developed over days to weeks (resembling GBS * respiratory failure and death in several patients. Systemic symptoms included nausea, vomiting, weight loss, abdominal distention, hepatomegaly, and lipoatrophy. Stavudine, Lamivudine and Efavirenz are most commonly used ARV agent. Muscle weakness worsened even after discontinuation of ARV therapy. Rapidly progressive sensorimotor polyneuropathy and myopathy observed. In recent years, a spectrum of metabolic and morphologic alterations has emerged among HIV-infected patients receiving HAART. Additionally, neurological syndromes, such as antiretroviral toxic neuropathy, have been clinically well characterized (Höke & Cornblath, 2004; Keswani et al., 2002). Diagnostic information find out by severe axonal neuropathy, increase Serum lactate level twice times than normal, decrease Serum bicarbonate and arterial pH level, increase serum CPK level. Electrophysiology; EMG-NCV: severe axonal neuropathy in most of the cases, demyelinating features may be seen admixed or in isolation and myopathic features may be noted. Nerve and Muscle Biopsy: Important in evaluating patients with HANWS. Mitochondrial studies with morphology assessment and mitochondrial DNA (mtDNA) quantification may be needed to further elucidate the role of mitochondrial toxicity in this syndrome Treatment: As was observed in this report, the antiretroviral most often associated with HANWS was stavudine. Avoiding stavudine or didanosine, the nucleosides with the highest association with mitochondrial toxicity, may be a satisfactory alternative in the long run. The treatment of HANWS is controversial and important since this is potentially a fatal syndrome. Our experience reinforces the recommendation that early interruption of HAART and clinical support is beneficial. Initiate systemic treatment for lactic acidosis syndrome and supportive treatment for the neurologic component in a monitored setting. Neuromuscular weakness - corticosteroids, intravenous immunoglobulins, vitamins (B1, B12), and plasmapheresis have been used (Luciano et al., 2003).

3.6. Toxoplasmosis

Toxoplasmosis is the leading cause of focal central nervous system (CNS) disease in AIDS. CNS toxoplasmosis in HIV-infected patients is usually a complication of the late phase of the disease. Toxoplasmosis has been an indicator disease for AIDS since the early days of the human immunodeficiency virus (HIV) epidemic (Horowitz et al., 1983; Luft et al., 1984). CNS toxoplasmosis begins with constitutional symptoms and headache. Later, confusion and drowsiness, seizures, focal weakness, and language disturbance develop. Without treatment, patients progress to coma in days to weeks. On physical examination, personality and mental status changes may be observed. Seizures, hemiparesis, hemianopia, aphasia, ataxia, and cranial nerve palsies may be evident. Occasionally, symptoms and signs of a radiculomyelopathy predominate. Serologic studies in patients with CNS toxoplasmosis may demonstrate rising titers of anti-toxoplasma immunoglobulin G (IgG) antibodies, CD4 counts < 100 cells mm^{-3} and CSF findings are non-specific. Detection of T.gondii DNA by PCR has only moderate sensitivity. MRI typically reveals multiple enhancing lesions with perifocal oedema and mass effect in the basal ganglia and gray white matter interface of the cerebral hemispheres. Any part of the brain can be affected, mostly solitary in appearance. Standard therapy consists of pyrimethamine, sulfadiazine, and folinic acid in combination. Trimethoprim-sulfamethoxazole (TMP-SMZ) can be used as an alternative regimen (Dedicoat et al., 2006). A Cochrane data base review failed to find a significant difference between standard therapy and TMP-SMZ. Clindamycin can be used in patients allergic to sulfa drugs. Effective antiretroviral therapy is equally important (Dedicoat et al., 2006; Fung et al., 1996; Bertschy et al., 2006; Behbahani et al., 1995). Most common cause of cerebral mass lesion, Sub acute course with fever, headache, confusion or cognitive disturbances with focal deficits, Seizures 24 – 29 %, rarely psychotic features. Imaging – Multiple mass lesions at grey – white junction & basal ganglia, CSF – Non specific, Antibody to T. Gondi, PCR recently developed.

3.7. AIDS related primary CNS lymphoma

A relationship between congenital or acquired immune deficiency (AIDS) and lymphoma was first recognised more than 30 years ago. An association between non-Hodgkin's lymphoma (NHL) and the acquired immune deficiency syndrome became evident in the early 1980s. Lymphoma occurring in the HIV-infected individual may be systemic, may primarily involve the central nervous system, or may be localised in the body cavities. Systemic lymphoma is the most common presentation, accounting for approximately 80% of all cases. The histology usually is diffuse large cell, immunoblastic, or small non-cleaved cell lymphoma. Primary CNS lymphoma accounts for approximately 20% of all cases. Most patients are profoundly immunosuppressed and typically have a CD4 lymphocyte count below 50/ml. Approximately two-thirds or more of them have AIDS-defining conditions prior to the development of primary CNS lymphoma (Gill et al., 1985; Goldstein, 1991). The lesions are typically few in number (1–3), large (2–4 cm), and contrast enhances approximately 50% of the time (Fine & Mayer 1993). Lesions are most common in the cerebrum, but also occur frequently in the cerebellum, basal ganglia and brain stem, and are nearly always found to be multifocal at autopsy (Loureiro et al., 1988; MacMahon et al., 1991). The lymphoma cells tend to be distributed along vascular channels as perivascular cuffs, are of B cell origin, display large cell and immunoblastic histologies. Subacute presentation with headache, impaired cognition, focal cerebral dysfunction. D/D – Toxoplasmosis, PML. Imaging – Multiple enhancing periventricular or subependymal lesions, CSF – EBV nucleic acid in CSF being studied. NHL are of higher grade and advanced stage. Response and tolerance to chemotherapy is poor. Systemic lymphoma in patients with HIV infection is a potentially curable disease, although the potential for cure is less than in immunocompetent individuals. Appropriate use of supportive care is an important component of therapy (Table 3) (Sparano, 2001).

Indication	Drug(s)
Primary infection prophylaxis	
Pneumocystis carinii, Toxoplasma	TMP-SMZ 1 DS QD
Oral and/or oesophageal candidiasis	Fluconazole 100 mg QD
MAI Complex (CD4 < 50/ul)	Azithromycin 1200 mg weekly
Secondary infection prophylaxis	
Herpes simplex infections	Acyclovir 400 mg BID or 200 mg TID
Cytomegalovirus infection	Ganciclovir 1 g TID
Mycobacterium-avium complex	Clarithromycin 500 mg BID plus ethambutol
	15 mg/kg QD, with or without rifabutin 300 mg QD
Toxoplasma gondii	Sulphadiazine 1–1.5 gm q6h, pyrimethamine 25–75 mg
	QD, Leucovorin 10–25 mg QD — QID
Cryptococcus neoformans	Fluconazole 200 mg QD
Salmonella bacteraemia	Ciprofloxacin 500 mg BID
Haematopoietic growth factors	
For selected patients in whom the risk of febrile neutropenia ≥ 40%	G-CSF 5 mcg/kg or GM-CSF 250 mcg/M² s.c. daily
	beginning after completion of chemotherapy and
	continue until neutrophil recovery
Antiretroviral agents	
Selecting patients for therapy	Follow NIH guidelines (http://www.hivatis.org)
Role of therapy in controlling malignancy	
Kaposi's sarcoma	Essential
Lymphoma	Unknown
Other tumours	Unknown
Factors influencing selection of agents	
May be used with myelosuppressive drugs	Didanosine, zalcitabine
Avoid with myelosuppressive drugs/regimens	Zidovudine
Avoid with neurotoxic drugs/regimens	Didanosine, zalcitabine, stavudine
May alter the metabolism of cytotoxic drugs metabolised by cytochrome p450 enzymes	All protease inhibitors and non-nucleoside RTIs

QD. Daily; TID, three times daily; BID, two times daily; QID, four times daily; s.c., subcutaneous; G CSF, granulocyte colony stimulating factor; GM,CSF, granulocyte-macrophage colony stimulating factor, NIH, national institute of health; RTIs, reserve transcript inhibitors.

Table 3. Suggested supportive care for the patient with HIV infection and lymphoma or other malignancies. European Journal of Cancer 37 (2001) 1296–1305

Appropriate supportive care and CNS prophylaxis might improve outcome. In patients with HIV infection, the differential diagnosis of a patient with focal brain lesions includes PCNSL, cerebral toxoplasmosis, and other infections. Focal brain lesions have also been described in conjunction with relapsed systemic lymphoma (Desai et al., 1999). A proposed algorithm for the diagnostic approach to a patient with HIV infection and focal brain lesions is shown in Fig. 3.

3.8. HIV related progressive multifocal leukoencephalopathy

Progressive Multifocal Leukoencephalopathy (PML) is a rare demyelinating disease (focal neurological disease & cognitive impairment) of the CNS caused by reactivation of JC virus (JCV) 1. Radiographic evidence of white matter disease with subcortical involvement – 'scalloped' appearance. CSF – Non specific. Primary infection occurs in childhood and the virus remains latent in the kidney or lymphoid organs thereafter. In the setting of cellular immunosuppression, the virus may spread to the central nervous system, leading to a lytic infection of oligodendrocytes and subsequent demyelination. Classically, PML was observed in patients with advanced HIV infection, lymphoproliferative disorders and transplant recipients. There is no specific treatment for PML, but the survival in HIV-infected PML patients has increased substantially during the last decade. Before the introduction of highly active antiretroviral therapy (HAART), only 10% patients with PML lived for more than a year. In contrast, recent studies have shown at least 50% one-year survival of HIV- infected PML patients (Falco et al., 2008; De Luca et al., 2008). However, the prognosis of PML associated with other immunosuppressive conditions remains poor. Immune recovery associated with HAART has resulted in a better prognosis for HIV-infected PML patients. The prompt institution of HAART in HIV infected PML patients is the most effective therapeutic approach in increasing survival in this group. Several studies have shown that PML survival increased from 10 to 50% in the last decade (Falco et al., 2008; De Luca et al., 2008; Cinque et al., 2003; Bamford et al., 1989; Du Pasquier et al., 2004; Koralnik et al., 2004; Gasnault et al., 2003; Antinori et al., 2003). In a recent study, JCV-peptide loaded dendritic cells from PML patients, HIV-infected individuals and healthy control subjects could elicit a strong cellular immune response mediated by CD8+ cytotoxic T lymphocytes cell response *in vitro* (Marzocchetti et al, 2009), which suggests that autologous dendritic cell-based immunotherapy could be a potential therapeutic option for PML.

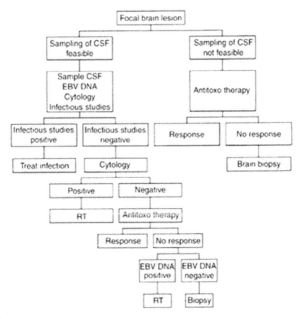

CSF, cerebrospinal fluid
Antitoxo, antitoxoplasmosis
RT, radiotherapy

Figure 3. Algorithm for management of HIV – infected individuals with focal brain lesions European Journal of Cancer 37 (2001) 1296–1305

3.9. Neurological approach to immunocompromized patients due to HIV-1

Central nervous system pathogens in specific immunocompromised-host (HIV-1) categories based upon presentation like Meningitis, Meningoencephalitis, and Encephalitis. Cryptococcal meningitis is seen in populations but cryptococcomas are much more frequent in the latter. Encephalitis and cerebral abscesses usually do not produce cerebrospinal fluid (CSF) changes unless the lesion communicates with the ventricular or subarachnoid spaces. Discrete white matter lesions have a narrower differential including calcineurin-induced demyelination usually in the posterior territory and progressive multifocal leukoencephalopathy (JC papova virus) which is characteristically nonenhancing and without mass effect. Meningoencephalitis due to Toxoplasma gondii continues to be the predominant pathogen in HIV-1 disease even with highly active antiretroviral therapy (HAART) exposure (Peter K. Linden, 2009).

3.10. Neurogenic manifestation of HIV infection in children

Twenty percent of children present with severe symptoms or die in infancy, Prognosis is related to: a) Greater inoculation of HIV b) Earlier infection with immature immune system c) Immune escape from mother. Asceptic Meningitis or Meningoencephalitis does not occur in infants. Acquired Microcephali, cerebral vasculopathy and basal ganglia, Calcification are unique in children. OIS are rare in children, here absolute CD_4T cell count less helpful. HIV-DNA PCR on peripheral blood lymphocytes can help to diagnosis. Avoid vaginal delivery, plan caesarean section and avoid breast feeding.

4. Markers for HIV progression

A combination of different markers is required to predict plasma human immunodeficiency virus type 1 (HIV-1) disease progression (Fahey et al., 1990; Saves et al., 2001). Levels of plasma HIV-1 RNA and CD4 + cell count are highly predictive of progression to AIDS or death (Hughes et al., 1997; Mellors et al., 1997; Saves et al., 2001). However, variations of these markers do not explain all variations of disease progression and the relative prognostic value of laboratory markers of HIV disease are not the same at different stages of the disease. Therefore the use of markers of immune activation has been suggested (Graham, 1996; Saves et al., 2001). CD4+ cell count (CD4) and RNA viral loads (RNA) are the two most commonly used prognostic markers of the clinical progression of HIV infection for HIV infection (Hammer et al., 2006; Gilks et al., 2006). Besides, there are various additional markers for HIV progression such as CD8+ cell count, anti-HIV antibodies, p24 antigen, hemoglobin concentration, platelet concentration as well as erythrocyte sedimentation rate (ESR). Various predictors for progression to AIDS among HIV-positive homosexual men have beed identified. These include low absolute number and/or percentage of CD4+ lymphocytes, low CD8+ cell count, low concentration of anti-HIV antibodies, p24 antigenaemia, decreased concentration of haemoglobin, increased titre of IgG antibody to cytomegalovirus, raised serum IgA and IgM values, raised concentrations in the serum of interleukin-2 receptor, neopterin and beta2-microglobulin (Gafa et al., 1993). Among these markers, the percentage of CD4+ cells was found to be the best predictor of HIV progression (Fahey et al., 1990), followed by serum concentrations of neopterin and beta2-microglobulin, IgA, interleukin-2 receptors and p24 antigen. Only a few studies have the predictive values of these serological markers which have been evaluated in cohorts of IVDUs (Gafa et al., 1993). De Wolf & Lange, (1993) observed that several laboratory markers become most noticeably established as predictors of progression from asymptomatic HIV-1 infection to AIDS: (1) Decline in antibody reactivity to HIV core proteins p24 and p17; (2) Appearance of persistent HIV-1 p24 antigenemia; (3) Declining numbers and percentages of peripheral blood CD4-positive lymphocytes; (4) Elevated serum beta2-microglobulin concentration and (4) Elevated serum and urine neopterin concentrations.

4.1. Immunological and virological markers

Based upon scientific literature, immunological and virological markers have been proven as prognostic indicators for progression of HIV disease. The most widely studied marker, the CD4 + lymphocyte count was found to be the best single indicator of the stage of the illness (Zeller et al., 1996). HIV infects CD4+ T lymphocytes selectively and causes the destruction of CD4+ T cells directly as well as indirectly leading to gradual loss of the CD4 T cell numbers in peripheral circulation. Hence, the CD4+ T cell counts are being used to monitor the disease progression in HIV infection, to decide the threshold for initiation of anti-retro viral therapy, to monitor the efficacy of Anti Retrroviral treatment and to initiate prophylactic treatment for opportunistic infections (OIs) (Atlh Nicholson, 1997; Pattanapanyasat & Thakat, 2005). Measuring the CD4+ lymphocytes count remains the most effective means of evaluating of the clinical prognosis of patients infected with Human Immunodeficiency Virus (HIV) (Stein et al., 1992). This measurement has been universally accepted as a uniform means for the clinical staging of patients infected with HIV and those progressing to AIDS (Levine et al., 2000) and for the determination of the commencement of antiretroviral therapy and for monitoring the response to antiretroviral therapy (Evans-Gilbert et al., 2004).

4.2. CD4+ cell count

CD4+ T lymphocyte play a central regulatory role in the immune response. The decrease in CD4+ T cell numbers can compromise the normal immune functions of the body. Hence, the number of CD4+ T cells in the circulation provides important information regarding the immune competence of an individual (Thakar et al., 2011). HIV primarily targets CD4 cells. As HIV disease progresses, CD4 cell counts decline, typically by about 30-100 cells/μl per year (depending on viral load), leaving a person increasingly vulnerable to infections and cancers. People with CD4 cell counts above 500 cells/μl generally have relatively normal immune function and are at low risk for opportunistic infections (Hammer et al., 2006). The clinical staging of HIV disease and the relative risk of developing opportunistic infections have historically relied on the CD4 cell count as the principle laboratory marker of immune status (Kleinman et al., 1998; Patton et al., 2003). HIV disease is commonly categorized on the basis of three levels of immunodeficiency: relative immune competence (CD4 cell count > 500/μl; ≥ 29%), early immune suppression (CD4 cell count between 200/μl and 500/ μl); 4%-28%) and severe immune suppression (CD4 cell count <200/μl and 500/ μl); <14%) (CDC, 1993).

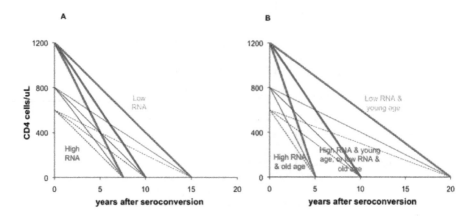

Figure 4. Schematic natural history model of HIV-1 replication driving rates of CD4 decline and clinical progression (Korenromp et al., 2009)

4.3. CD8+ cell count

There are two types of T cells carry the CD8 surface molecule: T-suppressor cells, which inhibit immune responses, and killer T cells (also known as cytotoxic T lymphocytes, or CTLs), which target and kill infected or cancerous cells. As with CD4 cells, a variety of factors can cause CD8 cell counts to fluctuate. CD8 cell counts typically rise over time in people with HIV, but (unlike CD4 cells) CD8 cell numbers do not independently predict disease progression, and their relation to immune status is not well understood (Vajpayee & Mohan 2011).

4.4. CD4 and CD8 cell percentage

Because absolute CD4 and CD8 cell counts are so variable, some physicians prefer to look at CD4 or CD8 cell percentages, the proportion of all lymphocytes that are CD4 or CD8 cells. Percentages are usually more stable over time than absolute counts. A normal CD4 cell percentage in a healthy person is about 30-60 per cent, while a normal CD8 cell percentage is 15-40 per cent (Taylor et al., 1989).

4.5. CD4/CD8 cell ratio

The CD4/CD8 cell ratio is calculated by dividing the CD4 cell count by the CD8 cell count. A normal CD4/CD8 cell ratio is about 0.9-3.0 or higher, there are at least 1-3 CD4 cells for every CD8 cell. In people with HIV this ratio may be much lower, with many more CD8 cells than CD4 cells (Giorgi, 1993).

4.6. HIV viral load

Viral load tests measure the amount of HIV RNA in the blood. The presence of RNA indicates that the virus is actively replicating or multiplying. Along with the CD4 cell count, viral load is one of the most valuable measures for predicting HIV disease progression and gauging when anti-HIV treatment is indicated and how well it is working. Viral load is expressed either as copies of RNA per milliliter of blood (copies/ml) or in terms of logs. A log change is an exponential or 10-fold change. For example, a change from 100 to 1,000 is a 1 log (10-fold) increase, while a change from 1,000,000 to 10,000 is a 2 log (100-fold) decrease. If the level of HIV is too low to be measured, viral load is said to be undetectable, or below the limit of quantification. However, undetectable viral load does not mean that HIV has been eradicated; people with undetectable viral load maintain a very low level of virus. Even when HIV is not detectable in the blood, it may be detectable in the semen, female genital secretions, cerebro-spinal fluid, tissues, and lymph nodes (Calmy et al., 2004; Petti et al., 2006; WHO, 2006). In primary HIV infection, patients may present with flu-like symptoms which usually occur during the first weeks of HIV-1 infection. It is associated with peak levels of HIV-1 RNA viremia, which subsequently declines until reaching a set point, where levels remain for months to years. Initial studies suggested that those with more symptomatic acute infection and longer duration of illness have faster rates of progression to AIDS (Koenig et al., 2006). A viral load of 100,000 copies/ml or more is considered high, while levels below 10,000 copies/ml are considered low. Research has consistently shown that higher viral loads are associated with more rapid HIV disease progression and an increased risk of death. Current U.S. HIV treatment guidelines (Koenig et al., 2006) recommend that people should consider starting treatment if their viral load is above 55,000 copies/ml (revised upward from 10,000 copies/ml in the previous guidelines). Importantly, most studies that have correlated viral load and HIV disease progression have been done in men; more recent research indicates that women may progress to AIDS at lower viral load levels, suggesting that the treatment threshold should perhaps be revised downward for women (Monica et al., 2002).

4.7. Beta2-microglobulin (β2-microglobulin)

β2-microglobulin is a low molecular weight protein that forms light chain of the class I major histocompatibility complex (MHC) which present on the surface of most somatic cells including T and B lymphocytes as well as macrophages (Cresswell et al., 1974; Lawlor et al., 1990; De Wolf and Lange 1991). It exhibits amino acid homology with the constant region of immunoglobins (Dar & Singh, 1999; Fauci & Lane, 1998; Quin & Benson, 1994). Circulating β_2-MG is generated during normal MHC I turnover (Lawlor et al., 1990) and thus is not specific to HIV-related cell death. Stimulation of lymphoid cells increases β2-microglobulinproduction. Elevated serum concentration are seen in renal failure, hepatitis, rheumatoid arthritis, myeloproliferative disorders, lymphoproliferative disorders, infectious mononucleosis, influenza A and cytomegalovirus infection (De wolf and Lange, 1991). Free β2-microglobin can be measured in both serum and urine and levels of urine β2-microglobin correlate with the degree of progression of HIV disease. It spikes in acute infection, declines and then rises during the infection. Levels of β2-microglobin are elevated in a variety of conditions charac-terized by lymphocyte activation and/ or lymphocyte destruction; *e.g.* lymphoproliferative syndromes, autoimmune diseases, viral infection and in patients with renal diseases. It can be measured in serum or plasma by using radio immunoassay radio immunoassay (RIA) or competivive ELISA based tests. B2-microglobin measurement has several advantages as a laboratory assay to help determine prognosis. By contrast with CD4 cell count which requires special procedures for specimen handling and processing, β2-microglobin can be measured with a serological assay and equipment available in many laboratories (Vajpayee & Mohan, 2011). Increased concentrations of this molecule are predictive of progression of HIV infection to AIDS (Moss et al., 1988).

4.8. Neopterin

Neopterin (6-D- erythrohydroxy-propylpterin) is a low molecular weight compound derived from an intermediate product of the *de novo* biosynthesis of tetrahydrobiopterin from guanosine triphosphate (GTP) (Dar & Singh, 1999; Fauci & Lane, 1998; Quin & Benson, 1994). It is an early marker of HIV infection. The levels rise further on progression from pre AIDS to clinical AIDS (Vajpayee & Mohan 2011). It is produced by macrophages after stimulation with gamma interferon. The levels have also been found to be associated with progression of HIV-1-related disease (Fuchs et al., 1988; Melmed et al., 1989; Kramer et al., 1989; De Wolf and Lange 1991) but the predictive value is slightly inferior to that of β2-microglobulin levels. Since neopterin levels are stimulated by HIV infection, measurement of neopterin levels can be useful in monitoring progression and evaluating antiviral therapy (Vajpayee & Mohan 2011).

4.9. Additional markers

Haematological manifestations of HIV infection are common and more frequently occur with progression of the disease. Therefore the complete blood count (CBC) is one of the important haematological parameters which need to checked for HIV patients. They may have low blood cell counts (cytopenias) due to chronic HIV infection or as a side effect of medications, particularly drugs that damage the bone marrow, where all blood cells are produced. Blood cell counts are typically reported as the number of cells per μl of blood (cells/μl) or as a percentage of all blood cells. HIV patients should be checked for CBC for every six months, and more often if they are experiencing symptoms or taking drugs associated with low blood cell counts (De Santis et al., 2011; Olayemi et al, 2008).

4.9.1. Red and white blood cells

Anemia is common in HIV positives. HIV itself and various OIs such as *Mycobacterium avium* complex (MAC) can affect red blood cells and their oxygen-carrying capacity (Volberding et al., 2003; Owiredu et al., 2011). People with HIV infection should be especially concerned with neutrophil and lymphocyte levels, in particular CD4 and CD8 cell counts. Neutrophils normally make up about 50-70 per cent of all white blood cells. Various anti-HIV drugs, OI medications [including ganciclovir (Cytovene), used to treat cytomegalovirus, or CMV], and cancer chemotherapies that suppress the bone marrow may lead to neutropenia (Firnhaber, 2010).

4.9.2. Platelets

Platelets are necessary for blood clotting. A normal platelet count is about 130,000-440,000 cells/μl. Low platelet counts (thrombocytopenia) - which can lead to easy bruising and excessive bleeding may be caused by certain drugs, autoimmune reactions, accelerated destruction by the spleen, or HIV disease itself (Torre & Pugliese, 2008). In 2012, Parinitha & Kulkarni study the haematological changes in HIV infection with correlation to CD4+ cell count. In their study, they found that among 250 patients studied, anaemia was seen in 210 (84%) of cases. Thrombocytopenia occurs in 45 (18%) cases. Majority of cases (70%) had CD4+ cell counts below 200 cells/mm3. Fifty-four cases (21.6%) had CD4 cell counts between 200 to 499 cells/mm3 and 21 (8.4%) cases had CD4 count more than 500 cells/mm3. In patients with CD4 counts less than 200 cells/mm3, anaemia was seen in 91.4% cases, leucopenia in 26.8% cases, lymphopenia in 80% cases and thrombocytopenia in 21.7% cases.

5. Summary

The prevalence of neurological associated with HIV-1 is estimated at 15 to 50% of patients (Dalakas et al., 1988; Cornblath et al., 1988; So et al., 1988; Monte et al., 1988; Gabbai et al., 1990). But it may be almost 100% when a pathological study is performed (Rizzuto et al., 1995; Gabbai et al., 1990). The etiology and pathogenesis of neurological disease associated with HIV infection is uncertain. It can be caused by the direct or indirect action of HIV and antibody production, or secondary to infections (CMV, MAC), toxic effects of certain drugs (isoniazid, vincristine, d4T, ddi, ddC), or nutritional deficiencies (vitamin B12) (Rizzuto et al., 1995; Dalakas et al., 1988; Figg et al., 1991; Browone et al., 1993; Pike et al., 1993; Abram et al., 1994; Kieburtz et al., 1991). HIV seropositive patients may be overlooked or misdiagnosed. A discerning clinical analysis may be helpful in the diagnosis of this common disease and several laboratory markers become most noticeably established as predictors of HIV-1 infection.

Author details

Rehana Basri* and Wan Mohamad Wan Majdiah

*Address all correspondence to: rehana@kk.usm.my

Neurology Craniofacial Sciences & Oral Biology, School of Dental Science, Universiti Sains, Malaysia

References

[1] Abeysena C. & De Silva HJ (2005). HIV in South Asia. Medicine, 33, 42-43

[2] Abrams DI, Goldman AI, Launer C, Korvick JA, Neaton JD, Crane LR, Grodesky M, Wakefield S, Muth K, Kornegay S (1994). A comparative trial of didano-sine or zalcitabine after treatment with zidovudine in patients with human immunodeficiency virus infection. *N Engl J Med* 330: 657-662.

[3] Alimonti JB., Ball T.B.& Fowke K.R. (2003). "Mechanisms of CD4+ T lymphocyte cell death in human immunodeficiency virus infection and AIDS". *J Gen Virol* 84: 1649–1661

[4] Antinori A, Cingolani A, Lorenzini P, Giancola ML, Uccella I, Bossolasco S, Grisetti S, Moretti F, Vigo B, Bongiovanni M, Del Grosso B, Arcidiacono MI, Fibbia GC,Mena M, Finazzi MG, Guaraldi G, Ammassari A, d'Arminio Monforte A, Cinque P, De Luca A. (2003). Clinical epidemiology and survival of progressive multifocal leukoencephalopathy in the era of highly active antiretroviral therapy: data from the Italian Registry Investigative Neuro AIDS (IRINA). *J Neurovirol* 9, Suppl 1:47–53.

[5] Artigas J., Grosse G. & Niedobitek F. (1990). Vacuolar myelopathy in AIDS: a morphologic analysis. *Pathol Res Pract* 186:228– 237

[6] Atlh Nicholson J.A. (1997). Revised guidelines for the performance of CD4+ T cell determinations in persons with human immunodeficiency virus infection. *Morb Mortal Wkly Rep* 46:41–29.

[7] Auger I, Thomas P, De Gruttola V, Morse D, Moore D, Williams R, Truman B, Lawrence CE. (1988). Incubation periods for paediatric AIDS patients. *Nature* 336: 575-77

[8] Bacchetti P. & Moss A.R. (1989). Incubation time of AIDS in San Francisco. *Nature* 338: 251-53

[9] Bamford J.M., Sandercock P.A., Warlow C.P. & Slattery J. (1989). Interobserver agreement for the assessment of handicap in stroke patients. *Stroke* 20(6): 828

[10] Behbahani R., Moshfeghi M. & Baxter J.D. (1995). Therapeutic approaches for AIDS-related toxoplasmosis. *Ann Pharmacother* 29 (7-8): 760-8.

[11] Browne MJ, Mayer KH, Chafee SB, Dudley MN, Posner MR, Steinberg SM, Graham KK, Geletko SM, Zinner SH, Denman SL. (1993). 2′,3′-didehydro-3′- deoxythymidine (d4T) in patients with AIDS and AIDS-related complex: a phase I trial. *J Infect Dis* 167: 21-29

[12] Calmy A., Klement E., Teck R., Berman D., Pecoul B. & Ferradini L. (2004). Simplifying and adapting antiretroviral treatment in resource-poor settings: a necessary step to scaling-up. *AIDS* 18: 2353–60

[13] Center for Disease Control and Prevention. (1993). Revised classification system for HIV infection and expanded surveillance case definition for AIDS among adolescents and adults. *MMWR Morb Mortal Wkly Rep* 1992; 41 (RR-17): 1-9.

[14] Cinque P., Koralnik I.J. & Clifford D.B. (2003). The evolving face of human immunodeficiency virus-related progressive multifocal leukoencephalopathy: defining a consensus terminology. *J Neurovirol* 9 Suppl 1:88–92

[15] Cornblath D.R. & McArthur J.C. (1988). Predominantly sensory neuropathy in patients with AIDS and AIDS-related complex. *Neurology* 38: 794-796

[16] Cresswell P, Springer T, Strominger JL, Turner MJ, Grey HM, Kubo RT. (1974). Immunological identity of the small subunit of HLA-A antigens and β2-microglobulin and its turnover on the cell membrane. *Proc Natl Acad Sci USA* 71: 2123-27

[17] Dalakas M.C. & Pezeshkpour G.H. (1988). Neuromuscular diseases associated with human immunodeficiency virus infection. *Ann Neurol* 23: 38-48

[18] Dal Pan, G.J., Glass J.D. & McArthur J.C. (1994). Clinicopathologic correlations of HIV-1-associated vacuolar myelopathy: an autopsybased case-control study. *Neurology* 44: 2159–64

[19] Dar L. & Singh Y.G.K. (1999). Laboratory tests for monitoring stage and progression of HIV infection. In HIV testing manual by NICD and NACO. New Delhi: CBS Publishers. 114–25

[20] Dedicoat M. & Livesley N. (2006). Management of toxoplasmic encephalitis in HIV-infected adults (with an emphasis on resource-poor settings). *Cochrane Database Syst Rev* 3:CD005420

[21] De la Monte SM, Gabuzda DH, Ho DD, Brown RH Jr, Hedley-Whyte ET, Schooley RT, Hirsch MS, Bhan AK. (1988). Peripheral neuropathy in the acquired immunodeficiency syndrome. *Ann Neurol* 23: 485-492

[22] Delpech V. & Gahagan J. (2009). The global epidemiology of HIV. *Medicine* 37: 317-20

[23] De Luca A, Ammassari A, Pezzotti P, Cinque P, Gasnault J, Berenguer J, Di Giambenedetto S, Cingolani A, Taoufik Y, Miralles P, Marra CM, Antinori A; Gesida. (2008).Cidofovir in addition to antiretroviral treatment is not effective for AIDS-associated progressive multifocal leukoencephalopathy: a multicohort analysis. *AIDS* 22(14): 1759–1767

[24] De Santis GC, Brunetta DM, Vilar FC, Brandão RA, de Albernaz Muniz RZ, de Lima GM, Amorelli-Chacel ME, Covas DT, Machado AA. (2011). Hematological abnormalities in HIV-infected patients. *Int J Infect* Dis.15: e808–11.

[25] Desai J., Mitnick R.J., Henry D.H., Llena J., Sparano J.A. (1999). Patterns of central nervous system recurrence in patients with systemic human immunodeficiency virus-associated non-Hodgkin's lymphoma. *Cancer* 86: 1840–1847

[26] Dorfman D., DiRocco A., Simpson D., Tagliati M., Tanners L. & Moise J. (1997). Oral methionine may improve neuropsychological function in patients with AIDS myelopathy: results of an open-label trial. *AIDS* 11(8): 1066-7

[27] Du Pasquier R.A., Kuroda M.J., Zheng Y., Jean-Jacques J., Letvin N.L., Koralnik I.J. (2004). A prospective study demonstrates an association between JC virus-specific cytotoxic T lymphocytes and the early control of progressive multifocal leukoencephalopathy. *Brain* 127(Pt 9): 1970–1978

[28] De Wolf F. & Lange J.M.A. (1991). Serologic and Immunologic Markers in the Course of HIV-1 Infection. Clinics in Dermatology: 1-11

[29] Evans-Gilbert T., Pierre R., Steel-Duncan J.C., Rodriguez B., Whorms S., Hambleton IR., Figueroa JP. & Christie CD. (2004). Antiretroviral drug therapy in HIV-infected Jamaican children. *West Indian Med J* 53(5):322–326

[30] Fahey JL, Taylor JM, Detels R, Hofmann B, Melmed R, Nishanian P, Giorgi JV. (1990). The prognostic value of cellular and serologic markers in infection with human immunodeficiency virus type I. *N Engl J Med* 322: 166-72

[31] Falcó V, Olmo M, del Saz SV, Guelar A, Santos JR, Gutiérrez M, Colomer D, Deig E, Mateo G, Montero M, Pedrol E, Podzamczer D, Domingo P, Llibre JM. (2008). Influence of HAART on the clinical course of HIV-1-infected patients with progressive multifocal leukoencephalopathy: results of an observational multicenter study. *J Acquir Immune Defic Syndr* 49(1):26–31.

[32] Fauci A.S. & Lane H.C. (1998). HIV disease: AIDS and related disorders. Chapter 308. In: Fauci AS, Braunwald E, Wilson JD, Martin JB, Kaspar DL, Hauser SL, Longo DL, editors. *Harrison's principles of internal medicine*. 14th ed. New York: Mc Graw Hill: 1816–8

[33] Figg W.D. (1991). Peripheral neuropathy in HIV patients after isoniazid therapy. *Drug Intell Clin Pharm* 25: 100-101

[34] Fine H.A. & Mayer R.J. (1993). Primary central nervous system lymphoma. *Ann Intern Med* 119: 1093–1104

[35] Firnhaber C., Smeaton L., Saukila N., Flanigan T., Gangakhedkar R. & Kumwenda J. et al. (2010). Comparisons of anemia, thrombocytopenia, and neutropenia at initiation of HIV antiretroviral therapy in Africa, Asia, and the Americas. *Int J Infect Dis* 14:e1088–92

[36] Fung H.B. & Kirschenbaum H.L (1996). Treatment regimens for patients with toxoplasmic encephalitis. *Clin Ther* 18(6): 1037-56; discussion 1036

[37] Fuchs D., Hansen A. & Reibnegger G. et al. (1988). Neopterin as a marker for activated cell-mediated immunity: Application in HIV infection. *Immunol Today* 9: 150-55

[38] Gabbai A.A, Schmidt B., Castelo A., Oliveira A.S.B, Lima J.G.C. (1990). Muscle biopsy in AIDS and ARC: analysis of 50 patients. *Muscle Nerve* 13,541-4

[39] Gafa S., Giudici M.G., Pezzotti P. & Rezza G. (1993). IgA as a marker of clinical progression among HIV-seropositive intravenous drug users. *Journal of Infection* 26: 33-38

[40] Gasnault J., Kahraman M., de Goer de Herve M.G., Durali D., Delfraissy J.F. & Taoufik Y. (2003). Critical role of JC virus-specific CD4 T-cell responses in preventing progressive multifocal leukoencephalopathy. *AIDS* 17(10):1443–49

[41] Gill P, Rarick M, Bernstein-Singer M, Harb M, Espina BM, Shaw V, Levine A. (1990). Treatment of advanced Kaposi's sarcoma using combination of bleomycin and vincristine. *Am J Clin Oncol* 13 : 315-319

[42] Gill P.S., Levine A.M., Meyer P.R. (1985). Primary central nervous system lymphoma in homosexual men: clinical, immunologic, and pathologic features. *Am J Med* 78 : 742–748

[43] Gilks CF, Crowley S, Ekpini R, Gove S, Perriens J, Souteyrand Y, Sutherland D, Vitoria M, Guerma T, De Cock K. (2006). The WHO public-health approach to antiretroviral treatment against HIV in resource-limited settings. *Lancet* 368: 505–10

[44] Giorgi J.V. (1993). Characterization of T lymphocyte subset alterations by flow cytometry in HIV disease. *Ann NY Acad Sci* 677:126–37.

[45] Goldstein J.D, Dickson D.W. & Moser F.G. (1991). Primary central nervous system lymphoma in acquired immunodeficiency syndrome: a clinical and pathologic study with results of treatment with radiation. *Cancer* 67: 2756–65

[46] Goldstick L., Mangybur T.I. & Bode R. (1985). Spinal cord degeneration in AIDS. *Neurology* 35: 103–6

[47] Griffin D.E. (1997). Cytokines in the brain during viral infection: clues to HIV-associated dementia. *J Clin Invest* 100: 2948–51

[48] Gray F., Gherardi R., Trotot P., Fenelon G. & Poirier J. (1990). Spinal cord lesions in the acquired immune deficiency syndrome (AIDS). *Neurosurg Rev* 13: 189–194

[49] Graham N.M.H. (1996). The role of immunologic and viral markers in predicting clinical outcome in HIV infection. *AIDS 10*: S21-S25

[50] Hammer SM, Saag MS, Schechter M, Montaner JS, Schooley RT, Jacobsen DM, Thompson MA, Carpenter CC, Fischl MA, Gazzard BG, Gatell JM, Hirsch MS,Katzenstein DA, Richman DD, Vella S, Yeni PG, Volberding PA; International AIDS Society-USA panel. (2006). Treatment for adult HIV infection: 2006 Recommendations of the International AIDS Society-USA panel. *JAMA* 296: 827–43

[51] Henin D., Smith T.W., De Girolami U, Sughayer M, Hauw J.J. (1992). Neuropathology of the spinal cord in the acquired immunodeficiency syndrome. *Hum Pathol* 23: 1106–14

[52] Höke A. & Cornblath. D.R. (2004). Peripheral neuropathies in human immunodeficiency virus infection. *Clin Neurophysiol* 57(Suppl): S195-S210

[53] Horowitz S.L , Bentson J.R., Benson F., Davos I., Pressman B. & Gottlieb M.S. (1983). CNS toxoplasmosis in acquired immunodeficiency syndrome. *Arch Neurol* 40: 649–52

[54] Hughes MD, Johnson VA, Hirsch MS, Bremer JW, Elbeik T, Erice A, Kuritzkes DR, Scott WA, Spector SA, Basgoz N, Fischl MA, D'Aquila RT. (1997). Monitoring plasma HIV-1 RNA levels in addition to CD4+ lymphocyte count improves assessment of antiretroviral therapeutic response: ACTG Protocol Virology Substudy Team. *Ann Int Med* 126: 929-938

[55] J.A. Sparano (2001). Clinical aspects and management of AIDS-related lymphoma. *European Journal of Cancer* 37, 1296–1305

[56] Phillips KD, Skelton WD, Hand GA (2004). Effect of acupuncture administered in a group setting on pain and subjective peripheral neuropathy in persons with human immunodeficiency virus disease. The journal of alternative and complementary medicine 10:3, 449–455.

[57] Keswani S.C., Pardo C.A., Cherry C.L., Höke A. & McArthur J.C. (2002). HIV-associated sensory neuropathies. *AIDS* 16: 2105-2117

[58] Kieburtz K.D., Giang D.W., Shiffer R.B., Vakil N. (1991). Abnormal vitamin B12 metabolism in human immunodeficiency virus infection: association with neurological dysfunction. *Arch Neurol* 48: 312-314

[59] Kleinman S, Busch MP, Hall L, Thomson R, Glynn S, Gallahan D, Ownby HE, Williams AE. (1998). False positive HIV-1 test results in a low-risk screening setting of voluntary blood donation. *JAMA* 280 (12): 1080-5

[60] Koralnik I.J. (2006). Progressive multifocal leukoencephalopathy revisited: Has the disease outgrown its name? *Ann Neurol* 60(2): 162–173

[61] Koralnik I.J , Schellingerhout D , Frosch M.P. (2004). Case records of the Massachusetts General Hospital. Weekly clinicopathological exercises. Case 14-2004. A 66-year-old man with progressive neurologic deficits. *N Engl J Med* 350 (18): 1882–1893

[62] Koenig S.P., Kuritzkes D.R., Hirsch M.S., Leandre F., Mukherjee J.S. & Farmer P.E. et al. (2006). Monitoring HIV treatment in developing countries. *BMJ* 332: 602–4

[63] Krämer A, Wiktor SZ, Fuchs D, Milstien S, Gail MH, Yellin FJ, Biggar RJ, Wachter H, Kaufman S, Blattner WA. (1989). Neopterin: A predictive marker of acquired immune deficiency syndrome in human immunodeficiency virus infection. *J Acquir Immune Defic Syndr* 2: 291-96

[64] Lawlor D.A., Zemmour J., Ennis P.D. & Parham P. (1990). Evolution of class-I MHC genes and proteins: from natural selection to thymic selection. *Annu Rev Immunol* 8: 23–63

[65] Lagakos S.W. & DeGruttola V. (1989). The conditional latency distribution of AIDS for persons infected by blood transfusions. *J Acquir Immune Defic Syndr* 2: 84-87

[66] Letendre SL, McCutchan JA, Childers ME, Woods SP, Lazzaretto D, Heaton RK, Grant I, Ellis RJ; HNRC Group. (2004). Enhancing antiretroviral therapy for human immunodeficiency virus cognitive disorders. *Ann Neurol* 56: 416–423

[67] Levine A.M., Seneviratne L., Espina B.M., Wohl A.R., Tulpule A., Nathwani B.N. &Gill PS. (2000). Evolving characteristics of AIDS-related lymphoma. *Blood* 96(13): 4084–90

[68] Liu Y, Tang XP, McArthur JC, Scott J, Gartner S. (2000). Analysis of human immunodeficiency virus type 1 gp160 sequences from a patient with HIV dementia: evidence for monocyte trafficking into brain. *J Neurovirol* 6: S70–S81

[69] Lui K.J, Lawrence D.N & Morgan W.M. (1988). A model-based estimate of the mean incubation period for AIDS in homosexual men. *Science* 240: 1333-35

[70] Loureiro C, Gill P.S., Meyer P.R., Rhodes R., Rarick M.U. & Levine A.M. (1988). Autopsy findings in AIDS-related lymphoma. *Cancer* 62: 735–739

[71] Luciano C.A., Pardo C.A. & McArthur J.C. (2003). Recent developments in the HIV neuropathies. *Curr Opin Neurol* 16: 403-9

[72] Luft B.J., Brooks R.G., Conley F.K., McCabe R.E., Remington J.S. (1984). Toxoplasmic encephalitis in patients with acquired immune deficiency syndrome, *JAMA* 252: 913–7

[73] Lui KJ, Darrow WW, Rutherford GW 3rd. (1988). A model-based estimate of the mean incubation period for AIDS in homosexual men. *Science* 240: 1333-35

[74] Mac Mahon, E.M, Glass, J.D, Hayward, S.D, Mann, R.B, Becker, P.S, Charache, P, McArthur, J.C, & Ambinder, R.F. (1991). Epstein Barr virus in AIDS-related primary central nervous system lymphoma. *Lancet* 338: 969–973

[75] Marzocchetti A, Lima M, Tompkins T, Kavanagh DG, Gandhi RT, O'Neill DW, Bhardwaj N, Koralnik IJ. (2009). Efficient in vitro expansion of JC virus-specific CD8(+) T-cell responses by JCV peptide-stimulated dendritic cells from patients with progressive multifocal leukoencephalopathy. *Virology* 383(2): 173–177

[76] McArthur JC, Haughey N, Gartner S, Conant K, Pardo C, Nath A, Sacktor N. (2003). Human immunodeficiency virus-associated dementia: an evolving disease. *J Neurovirol* 9: 205–221

[77] Medley G.F., Anderson R.M., Cox D.R. & Billard L. (1987). Incubation period of AIDS in patients infected via blood transfusion. *Nature* 328: 719-21

[78] Mellors JW, Muñoz A, Giorgi JV, Margolick JB, Tassoni CJ, Gupta P, Kingsley LA, Todd JA, Saah AJ, Detels R, Phair JP, Rinaldo CR Jr. (1997). Plasma viral load and CD4+ lymphocyte as prognostic markers of HIV-1 infection. *Ann Int Med* 126: 946-954

[79] Melmed RN, Taylor JM, Detels R, Bozorgmehri M, Fahey JL.Melmed. (1989). Serum neopterin changes in HIV-infected subjects: indicator of significant pathology CD4 T cell changes and the development of AIDS. *J Acquire Immune Defic Syndr* 2: 70-76

[80] Mirsattari S.M., Power C. & Nath A. (1998). Parkinsonism with HIV infection. *Mov Disord* 13: 684–9

[81] Monica G., Peter B., Paolo M., Thomas C.Q., Fulvia V. & Ruth M.G. (2002). Does patient sex affect human immunodeficiency virus levels? *Clin Infect Dis* 35:313–22

[82] Moss AR, Bacchetti P, Osmond D, Krampf W, Chaisson RE, Stites D, Wilber J, Allain JP, Carlson J. (1988). Seropositivity for HIV and the development of AIDS or AIDS related condition: three year follow up of the San Francisco General Hospital cohort. *Br Med J* 296: 745–50

[83] Navia B.A., Cho E.S., Petito C.K, Price RW. (1986). The AIDS dementia complex: II. Neuropathology. *Ann Neurol* 19: 525–35

[84]   Norton G.R., Sweeney J., Marriott D., Law M.G., Brew B.J. (1996). Association between
       HIV distal symmetric polyneuropathy and *Mycobacterium avium* complex infection. J
       Neurol Neurosurg

[85]   Olayemi E., Awodu O.A. & Bazuaye G.N. (2008). Autoimmune hemolytic anemia in
       HIV-infected patients: a hospital based study. *Ann Afr Med*

[86]   Owiredu W.K., Quaye L., Amidu N. & Addai-Mensah O. (2011). Prevalence of anaemia
       and immunological markers among ghanaian HAART-naïve HIV-patients and those
       on HAART. *Afr Health Sci* 11: 2–15

[87]   Petito C.K, Navia B.A, Cho E.S, Jordan BD, George DC, Price RW (1985). Vacuolar
       myelopathy pathologically resembling subacute combined degeneration in patients
       with the acquired immunodeficiency syndrome. *N Engl J Med* 312: 874–879

[88]   Peter K.L. (2009). Approach to the Immunocompromised Host with Infection in the
       Intensive Care Unit. *Infect Dis Clin N Am* 23 535–556.

[89]   Pike I.M. & Nicaise C. (1993). The didanosine expanded access program: safety analysis.
       Clin Infect Dis 16, S63-S68

[90]   Parinithas S. & Kulkarni M. (2012). Haematological changes in HIV infection with
       correlation to CD4 cell count. *Australas Med J* 5(3): 157-62

[91]   Patton LL. (2003). HIV disease. *Dent Clin N Am* 47: 467-492

[92]   Pattanapanyasat K. & Thakar MR. (2005). CD4+ T cell count as a tool to monitor HIV
       progression & anti-retroviral therapy. *Indian J Med Res* 121: 539–49

[93]   Peters P.J., Kilmarx P.H.& Mastro T.D. (2008). AIDS: Global Epidemiology. Encyclo-
       pedia of Virology (3rd Edition): 56-68

[94]   Petti C.A., Polage C.R., Quinn T.C., Ronald A.R. & Sande M.A. (2006). Laboratory
       medicine in Africa: a barrier to effective health care. *Clin Infect Dis* 42:377–82

[95]   Quinn T.C. (1990). The Epidemiology of the human immunodeficiency virus. *Annals of
       Emergency Medicine* 19: 225-32

[96]   Quin J.W. & Benson E.M. (1994). It is HIV: Immediate and long term plans. Chapter 24.
       In: Stewart G, editor. Could it be HIV? 2nd ed. Sydney, Australia: Australasian medical
       publishing company Ltd; 66–9

[97]   Rizzuto N, Cavallaro T, Monaco S, Morbin M, Bonetti B, Ferrari S, Galiazzo-Rizzuto S,
       Zanette G, Bertolasi L. (1995). Role of HIV in the pathogenesis of distal symmetrical
       peripheral neuropathy. *Acta Neuropathol* (Berl) 90: 244-50

[98]   Simpson D.M. & Tagliati M. (1995). Nucleoside analogue-associated peripheral
       neuropathy in human immunodeficiency virus infections. *J Acquir Immune Def Syndr
       Hum Retrovirol* 9, 153-161

[99] Snider WD., Simpson DM., Nielsen S., Gold JW., Metroka CE., Posner JB. (1983). Neurological complications of acquired immune deficiency syndrome: analysis of 50 patients," *Ann Neurol* 14: 403-418.

[100] So Y.T., Holtzman D.M., Abrams D.I. & Olney R.K. (1988). Peripheral neuropathy associated with acquired immunodeficiency syndrome: prevalence and clinical features from a population-based survey. *Arch Neurol* 45: 945-48

[101] Saves M., Morlat P., Chene G., Peuchant E., Pellegrin I, Bonnet SF., Bernard N., Lacoste D., Salamon R. & Beylot J. (2001). Prognostic value of plasma markers of immune activation in patients with advanced HIV disease treated by combination antiretroviral therapy. *Clinical Immunology* Vol 99. (3): 347-352.

[102] Sparano J.A (2001). Clinical aspects and management of AIDS-related lymphoma European Journal of Cancer 37: 1296–1305

[103] Stein D.S., Korvick J.K. & Vermund SH. (1992). CD4+ Lymphocyte cell enumeration for prediction of clinical course of human immunodeficiency virus disease: a review. *J Infect Dis* 165: 352–363

[104] Tan S.V., Guiloff R.J. & Scaravilli F. (1995). AIDS-associated vacuolar myelopathy: a morphometric study. *Brain* 118: 1247–61

[105] Taylor J.M.G., Fahey J.L., Detels R. & Giorgi J.V. (1989). CD4 percentage, CD4 number, and CD4:CD8 ratio in HIV infection: Which to choose and how to use. *J Acquir Immune Defic Syndr* 2:114–24

[106] Thakar MR, Abraham PR, Arora S, Balakrishnan P, Bandyopadhyay B, Joshi AA, Devi KR, Vasanthapuram R, Vajpayee M, Desai A, Mohanakrishnan J, Narain K, Ray K, Patil SS, Singh R, Singla A, Paranjape RS. (2011). Establishment of reference CD4+ T cell values for adult Indian population. *AIDS Res Ther* 8: 35.

[107] Torre D. & Pugliese A. (2008). Platelets and HIV-1 infection: old and new aspects. *Curr HIV Res* 6: 411–8

[108] Vajpayee M. & Mohan T. (2011). Current practices in laboratory monitoring of HIV infection. *Indian J Med Res* 134 (6): 801-22

[109] Volberding P.A., Baker K.R. & Levine A.M. (2003). Human immunodeficiency virus hematology. *Haematol Am Soc Hematol Educ Program*: 294–313

[110] World Health Organization : Geneva. (2006). Antiretroviral therapy for HIV infection in adults and adolescents in resource-limited settings: towards universal access.

[111] Zeller J.M., McCain N.L. & Swanson B. (1996). *Journal of the Association of Nurses in AIDS care* Vol 7. Issue 1: 15-17

[112] Zanetti C, Manzano GM, Gabbai AA (2004). The frequency of peripheral neuropathy in a group of HIV positive patients in brazil. *Arq Neuropsiquiatr* 62(2-A): 253-256

Chapter 8

Human Immunodeficiency Virus Infection and Co-Morbid Mental Distress

Peter J. Chipimo and Knut Fylkesnes

Additional information is available at the end of the chapter

1. Introduction

HIV/AIDS is probably the most challenging and pressing health issue of our time. Current estimates show that over 40million people are now living with HIV. Despite the availability of antiretroviral therapy, the provision of this treatment continues to pose a big challenge for various reasons. Globally, of the 6 million people requiring treatment, only 8% receive it – with considerable geographical inequity ie. High income countries vs. low income countries. Despite understanding the risk factors for HIV infection, the incidence of new HIV cases has not reduced at an acceptable rate. An unprecedented number of people still have no access to treatment and continue to die from HIV related problems. This has brought about devastating social and economic consequences at country level, family level and at personal level. A considerable number of individuals suffer from mental disorders resulting from being HIV infected. Independently, mental disorders make a substantial independent contribution to the burden of disease worldwide. The recognition of mental disorders as a major contributor to the global burden of disease has led to an increase in the demand for the inclusion of mental health services in primary health care as well as in community-based health surveys in order to improve screening, diagnosis and treatment of mental distress. It is estimated that, neuropsychiatric conditions account for up to 15% of all disability-adjusted life-years, and up to 30% of those attributable to non-communicable diseases. Neuropsychiatric disorders also account for 1.2 million deaths every year. These figures are most likely underestimated as official statistics especially in low and middle income countries are scanty and unreliable. In sub-Saharan Africa, it has been reported that 20–30% of primary health care centre attendees present with depressive symptoms as the first or secondary reason for seeking medical care. A study conducted in Tanzania revealed a 41.6% prevalence of depressive symptoms among primary health care patients while a similar study in Uganda reported a 20–30% prevalence of psychological disorders and depression among health care seekers. These research findings have also shown heightened risk for common mental disorders among the women i.e. a female to male ratio of 1.5–2.0. Other determinants have been found to include low socioeconomic position indicated by poor access to resources, unemployment and low educational attainment. It has also been shown to be higher among those with poor socio-support networks such as the unmarried, widowed and divorced. Mental disorders interact with many other health conditions, communicable and non-communicable. They commonly affect individuals with medical conditions and have been associated with adverse impacts on several measures of morbidity and mortality. Depressed patients have been shown to have worse physical, social and overall health than other patients. Of particular interest to this chapter is the interaction between HIV and mental distress

2. HIV and mental distress

Early stages of HIV epidemic

In the early stages of the HIV epidemic, the individuals who were affected did not know that their behaviour predisposed them to a potentially fatal disease. The epidemic also mushroomed at the time of a liberal and tolerant culture and dis-inhibited sexual restraint. Hence multiple sexual partners spread the epidemic in communities where these behaviours were more rampant. Intravenous drug use also contributed to the early spread of the epidemic. In the low and middle income countries, factors surrounding poor socio-economic position (poor education and low income) and inability to negotiate for condom use due to the disparity between the male and female gender have emerged as stronger predictors. Several early and recent epidemiologic studies elucidated these risk factors and more concerted effort was placed on public education directed at prevention. Other more recent innovations directed at rolling-back HIV infection have included massive male circumcision campaigns, innovation directed at the girl child to reduce early teenage pregnancies and early marriages and the introduction of Highly Active Anti-Retroviral Therapy (HAART). Recently efforts have been directed at the role mental distress plays in determining acquisition of HIV infection, initial individual's reaction and post-infection adaptation. Further poor mental health has been associated with subsequent development of AIDS.

Mental distress

Mental distress in the context of this book chapter refers to a term used by users of mental health services as well as some mental health practitioners in describing a wide array of experiences of a patient's life that commonly manifest as somatic symptoms and held to be out of the ordinary, distressing, troubling or confusing for the patient, without actually being ill in the medical sense. Chipimo and Fylkesnes identified some of the common causes of mental distress in a study conducted among primary health care centers in Zambia. (Table 1)

Category of factor	Frequency	Symptoms/comments
Worries about money	51	Concerns about rent, day-to-day living, school fees
Problems of the mind	47	Recurrent headaches, sleeplessness, unhappiness, trouble thinking, loss of appetite, night mares
Unknown cause of symptoms	32	Most common among informants not acknowledging symptoms as an illness or as mental distress, suggested witchcraft
Relationship with spouse and family members	26	Commonest among women, included crying more than usual, unhappiness, headaches, sleeplessness.
Ill health	24	Sleeplessness, daily life suffering, inability to play useful role in life, tiredness
Low self-esteem	16	Worthlessness, loss of interest, unhappiness, crying more than usual, difficulty enjoying daily activities, experience of stigma
Recent life events	6	Bereavement, divorces, newly diagnosed with chronic disease including HIV. Included symptoms of restlessness, sleeplessness, trouble thinking, headache, unhappiness

Table 1. Factors associated with Mental Distress as identified by the informants (Chipimo & Fylkesnes, 2011)

The term mental distress is seen by users of mental health services as less stigmatizing as it fits better with the social model of disability, since everyone experiences mental distress at one time or the other. The other synonym is psychological distress. The term is also often preferred as they feel it better captures the uniqueness and personal nature of their experiences. Mental distress is often thought of as being a concept with a wider scope than the regularly used traditional term, mental illness. The later being a specific set of symptoms medically defined in psychiatry, for example: Mania, schizophrenia, anxiety disorders, depression etc. Difficult life situations such as: poor social-support structures, bereavement, stress, poor sleep, drug and alcohol abuse can induce mental distress. These inducers could be temporary and resolve without further medical intervention. However individuals who have protracted episodes and endure such symptoms longer are more likely to be diagnosed with mental illness. This definition is not without controversy and often these terms are used interchangeably.

Double tragedy

Mental distress has been recognised as a crucial factor to some individual's ability to modify their behaviour to prevent HIV infection. With effective treatment options now available, care for HIV has become more dynamic and has transformed the HIV squeal from terminal care to chronic care. This further complicates the scenario as mental disorders have further been recognised as severely complicating treatment. These factors work in tandem with HIV causing direct damage on the brain, creating turmoil in the lives of the infected and further exacerbates mental disorders. Further the mental disorders reduce the individual's ability to effectively change behaviour thus increasing the risk of infection and morbidity. Published literature showing that individuals with pre-existing mental disorders are at increased risk for contracting HIV/AIDS has been largely indirect. However consistent reports from several countries have suggested that individuals with mental disorders have a higher sero-prevalence for HIV/AIDS and that mental distress generally precedes HIV infection. This is valid given that significant risk of HIV transmission exists within an individual's network. Frequencies of 30-60% behavioural risk factors that have been identified among individuals with mental distress include: high rates of unprotected sexual contact, poor adherence to condom use and injection-drug abuse. In a study conducted among gay men with depressive symptoms, use of alcohol and drugs before sex were identified as independent predictors for sero-conversion. In a systematic review comparing an HIV sero-positive group and HIV sero-negative control group, the prevalence of depression in the sero-positive group was two times higher than in the sero-negative (OR 2.0, 95% CI 1.3-3.0).

3. Aetiology of HIV related mental distress

HIV related mental distress can occur in multiple phases in which premorbid psychological and social adjustment issues play a vital role. Additionally other social factors such as household income, culture, religion and family circumstances also influence and can alter an individual's reaction to a diagnosis of HIV and subsequent adaptation to living with the diagnosis. The same factors have also been shown to influence and pose high risk of being infected With HIV. Put together all these factors singly or severally affect the clinical presentation and management of HIV patients. It is as such imperative that these factors are addressed and assessed in both the Voluntary-Counselling-and-Testing (VCT) and in the pre-HAART assessment. A self-perpetuating cycle (figure 1) of increasing morbidity appears to occur between HIV and mental distress; HIV infection leads to development of mental distress and/or pre-existing mental distress predispose to HIV infection. In their study, Chipimo and Fylkesnes (2009) showed that HIV infection has both a direct and indirect effects on genesis of mental distress.

Direct effect

HIV infection has been known to affect all other organ systems in the human body and is said to have replaced syphilis as the "great imitator" in the central nervous system (CNS) and almost any psychiatric or neurological presentation is possible. The CNS is the second most commonly affected organ in patients with AIDS. HIV can cause direct organic brain tissue damage thus leading to the development of mental disorders (Psychotic and non-psychotic). Virtually any mental disorder is possible. Among the most notable are depression and anxiety, personality disorders and dementia. The mechanisms explaining the development of these mental disorders are largely poorly understood but the presence of HIV-1-binding sites in the brain (chemokine receptors) allows HIV-1 to infect macrophages and microglia. It is however thought that it does not affect neurons, although neurons are injured and die by apoptosis. The pathway to neuronal injury is thought to be through release of macrophage, microglial and astrocyte toxins alongside the contribution of direct injury on the neurons by viral proteins. These toxins overstimulate neurons, resulting in the formation of free radicals and excitotoxicity, similar to other neurodegenerative diseases.

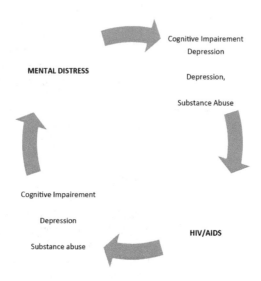

Figure 1. Self-perpetuating cycle of increasing morbidity: HIV/AIDS and Mental Distress (Chipimo, 2011)

Many HIV related opportunistic infections may involve the brain and lead to mental disorders. The four most frequent conditions are toxoplasmosis, progressive multifocal leukoencephalopathy (PML), cryptococcosis and cytomegalovirus infection. Although the incidence of these infections among patients with AIDS has decreased in the past years as a consequence of the introduction of highly active antiretroviral therapy (HAART), they remain a major cause of morbidity and mortality in this patient group. However, highly active antiretroviral drugs themselves such as, Zidovudine, Didanosine and Effervirenz have been associated with development of manic episodes

Indirect effect

Chipimo and Fylkesnes (2009) studied the relationship between HIV and mental distress in a population with high prevalence of HIV infection and low awareness of own HIV sero-status. In this study structural equation modeling (SEM) was used to establish the relationship between HIV infection and mental distress using maximum likelihood ratio as the method of estimation. The model indicated that underlying factors such as residence (rural or urban), level of education, marital status and age were inter-correlated as determinants for mental distress. Further Mental distress was found to be directly related to self-perceived risk and worry about being HIV infected, HIVsero-status and self-rated health. Further indirect inter-relationships were also found between self-rated health, self-perceived risk and worry about being HIV infected, and the underlying factors, namely age, residence, socio-economic position and education. Therefore self-rated health and self-perceived risk and worry about being HIV infected appear to be important mediators between underlying factors and mental distress. They are also important mediators between HIV status and mental distress. The results suggest that HIV infection has a substantial effect on mental distress both directly and indirectly. This effect was mediated through self-perceptions of health status, found to capture changes in health perceptions related to HIV, and self-perceived risk and worry of actually being HIV infected.

4. Prevalence of HIV related mental distress

Prevalence studies conducted world over have shown that when compared to the general population, mental disorders where considerably higher among the HIV infected individuals. However most of these studies have been conducted in the high income countries were the disease burden is relatively low and confined to selected groups for example Injection drug users and Homosexuals. Similar data in sub-Saharan Africa, where the HIV epidemic has its worse impact is limited. Therefore, given that mental disorders manifest in the majority of HIV infected individuals over the course of the illness, a simple assumption would then be that the prevalence reported in published studies represent an underestimate of the actual prevalence. A meta-analytic study identified 13 studies on mental disorders and HIV infection in low and middle income countries. The prevalence of mental disorders varied widely among these studies. Most of the studies done in Africa with HIV positive participants have shown differing but high percentages of mental distress, for example, Orange free state, South Africa 40%, rural Ethiopia 14% and Botswana 28%. In a study done in Zambia, Chipimo and Fylkesnes (2009) found a 13% prevalence of mental distress within the general population with a 2.0 higher odds ratio among the HIV infected. In Uganda, Musisi et. al. (2006) showed a 42% prevalence of depression among HIV infected individuals while in another study, Musisi & Kinyanda reported a prevalence of 41% among HIV infected adolenscents.

5. Presentation of HIV related mental distress

Diagnosis of mental disorders in HIV infection is a relatively rarely made diagnosis in sub-Saharan Africa. Studies have reported that physicians tend to be oblivious to psychological problems in HIV in the presence of a physical ailment. Further, the clinical presentation of mental distress in HIV infection presents a diagnostic challenge. This is often because the clinical Indictors of mental disorders are often masked by the symptoms of HIV infection. It is also a challenge for health care providers to distinguish between mental distress and grief. This calls for careful history taking that probes for previous history of mental disorders in the patient, suicide attempts, family history of mental illness, poor social support structures and a history of recent adverse events (deaths in family, physical violence, divorce, stigma).

Symptoms

Several studies have shown that mental distress often presents as somatisation. In a population based survey, Chipimo and Fylkesnes (2009) reported that the most frequently reported symptoms among the HIV infected were:

1. difficulty enjoying life,
2. feeling that their daily life was suffering,
3. poor sleep
4. low energy levels.

Among patients attending Primary Health Care, the most commonly reported symptoms observed by Chipimo and Fylkesnes (2010) were:

1. feelings of unhappiness,
2. loss of interest,
3. inability to enjoy daily life,
4. poor sleep
5. frequent headaches

Women reported these symptoms more than men in both studies. Musisi and Akena (2009) reported similar battery of symptoms and further added that, an otherwise asymptomatic HIV infected individual presenting with symptoms of fatigue and insomnia should be assessed for severe depression. These and other more pathognomonic symptoms put together allow clinicians to make a diagnosis of a full blown psychiatric disorder. The recognised HIV related psychiatric disorders are:

1. Anxiety disorders and depression
2. Psychotic disorder (Primary or secondary)
3. HIV-related Mania
4. HIV-related Dementia
5. HIV-related Delirium
6. Drug abuse ie. Substance and Alcohol abuse

6. Impact of HIV related mental distress on course and prognosis

There is a general lack of reported/ published follow-up studies on HIV related mental distress. However left untreated mental distress has an effect on the cell mediated immunity, where it causes impairments in T-cell mediated functions, reduced natural-killer cell counts and cytotoxicity. Depression in particular, has reproducibly been associated with decreased numbers and altered functioning of natural killer lymphocytes. It can also lead to an increase in activated CD8 T lymphocytes and viral load. By so doing mental distress can predict the onset and progression of both physical and social disability in HIV infection. Further, Co-morbid mental distress can delay health seeking hence reducing the likelihood of diagnosis and so can affect treatment and outcome in HIV infection. They may also adversely affect adherence to medication and activities to prevent disease and promote health.

7. Management

Mental disorders episodes are known to cluster around specific times in the course of the illness, such as, the period of diagnosis of HIV, period when the infected individual starts declining in health or the period in the early stages of HIV dementia. However, an episode of mental distress can occur at any point in the course of the illness. In the early stages social support alone can suffice alongside psychotherapy. However, in the later stages anti-depressants such as Imipramine or Amitriptyline can be used. Selective serotonin re-uptake inhibitors such as Fluoxetine may also be prescribed.

However the mainstay of management should fall around the time of diagnosis with adequate pre and post testing counseling surrounding the HIV test. The HIV counseling process should also be optimized to conditions that allow for higher acceptability of the counseling process. A Clinical trial study conducted in Zambia showed higher acceptability for Home-based-Voluntary-Counseling and testing as opposed to facility based counseling. Such innovative means of facilitating the counseling process will by induction lead to better acceptance of the HIV sero-status thus preventing subsequent maladjustment disorders. This has been shown in literature to reduce the risk of suicide at the initial diagnosis. Additionally follow-up counseling at every stage in the disease process emphasizing safer sex should be promoted alongside care giver support. This support should especially be extended to the most vulnerable; the women, children, orphans and those of low socio-economic position in society.

8. Conclusion

Mental disorders are common place in HIV infection and potentiate the course, progression and prognosis of the HIV disease process. The direct and indirect impact of HIV on the infected individual has conversely also been associated with mental distress episodes. Mental disorder and HIV/AIDS also have a lot of socio-demographic factors in common that have been attributed to each of their development. Therefore, a combination of these two disease entities leads to devastating morbidity and mortality, especially in the most affected communities. This thus emphasizes the need for prompt screening, diagnosis and treatment of mental distress in HIV infection.

Author details

Peter J. Chipimo[1,2] and Knut Fylkesnes[1]

1 University of Bergen, Faculty of Medicine, Centre for International Health, Norway

2 University of Zambia, School of Medicine, Department of Public Health, Zambia

References

[1] Bock PJ, Markovitz D. Infection with HIV-2. AIDS. 2001;15(Suppl 5):S35-45.

[2] Chipimo P.J. Fylkesnes K, Mental distress in the general population in Zambia: Impact of HIV and social factors: BMC Public Health. 2009; 9: 298. http://www.ncbi.nlm.nih.gov/pmc/articles/PMC2744699/

[3] Chipimo Peter J, Mental health in the era of HIV. Investigating mental distress, its determinants, conceptual models and the impact of HIV in Zambia. BORA-UiB 2011 http://hdl.handle.net/1956/4882

[4] Chipimo PJ, Fylkesnes K. Comparative validity of screening instruments for Mental Distress in Zambia. Clinical practice & Epidemiology in Mental Health. 2010;6:4-15.

[5] Chipimo PJ, Tuba M, Fylkesnes K, Conceptual models for Mental Distress among HIV infected and uninfected: A contribution to clinical practice and research in primary health-care centers in Zambia. BMC Health Services Research 2011; 11:7 1-12

[6] Chipimo, Peter Jay: Mental Distress and the Impact of HIV: Data from a Population-Based Survey in Zambia, Master thesis (2007) http://www.uib.no/cih/en/research/cih-master-theses

[7] Department of Health and Human Services (Ed). A Pocket Guide to Adult HIV/AIDS Treament January edition 2005

[8] DeVellis RF. Scale Development: Theory and Application. London: SAGE Publications; 2003.

[9] Escobar JI, Waitzkin H, Silver RC, Gara M, Holman A. A bridged somatization: a study in primary care. Psychosom Med. 1998;60:466-72.

[10] Gottlinger HG. The HIV-1 assembly machine. AIDS. 2001;15(Suppl 5):S13-20.

[11] Jenkins R. Sex differences in minor psychiatric morbidity: a survey of a homogeneous population. Social Science and Medicine. 1985;20(9):887-99.

[12] Kigozi FN, Flisher AJ, Lund C, Funk M, Banda M, Bhana A, et al. Mental health policy development and implementation in four African Conutries. Journal of health psychology. 2007;12(3):505-16.

[13] Kitahata MM, Gange SJ, Abraham AG, et al. Effect of early verses defered anti-retro-viral therapy for HIV on survival. N Engl Med. 2009;360(18):1815-26.

[14] Kroenke K, Spitzer RL, Williams JB, et al. Physical symptoms in primary care: Predictors of psychiatric disorders and functional impairement. Arch Fam Med. 1994;3:774-9.

[15] Kuehner C. Gender diffferences in unipolar depression: an update of epidemiological findings and possible explanations. Acta Psychiatr Scand. 2003;108:163-74.

[16] Maier W, Gansicke M, Gater R, Rezaki M, Tiemens B, Urzua RF. Gender differences in the prevalence of depression: A survey in primary care. J Affect Disord. 1999;53:241-52.

[17] Mathers CD, Loncar D. Projections of global mortality and burden of disease from 2002 to 2030. Plos Med. 2006;3(e442).

[18] McCaffery JM, Frasure-Smith N, Dude MP, et al. Common genetic vulnerability to depressive symptoms and coronary artery disease: a review and development of candidate genes related to inflamation and serotonin. Psychosom Med. 2006;68:187-200.

[19] Murray CJL, Lopez AD, et al. The global burden of disease and injuries series: A comprehensive assessment of Mortality and disability, Injuries and Risk factors 1990 and projected to 2020. Volume 1: Cambridge, MA; 1996.

[20] Ngoma MC, Prince M, Mann A. Common mental disorders among those attending primary health clinics and traditional healers in urban Tanzania. Br J Psychiatry. 2003;183:349-55.

[21] Ovuga EBL, Boardman A, Oluka GAO. Traditional healers and mental illness in Uganda. Psychiatric Bull. 1999;23:276-9.

[22] Palella FJ, Delaney KM, Moorman AC, Loveless MO, Fuhrer J, Satten GA, et al. Declining morbidity and mortality among patients with advanced human immunodeficiency virus infection. N Engl Med. 1998;338(13):853-60.

[23] Patel V, Abas M, Broadhead J, Todd CH, Reeler AP. Depression in developing countries: Lessons from Zimbabwe. BMJ. 2001;322(482).

[24] Rachlis AR, Zarowny DP. Guidelines for anti-retroviral therapy for HIV infection. Canadian HIV trials Network Antiretroviral Working Group. CMAJ. 1998;158(4): 496-505.

[25] Sax PE, Baden LR. When to start anti-retroviral therapy- ready when you are? N Engl Med. 2009;360(18):1897-9.

[26] Saz P, Dewey ME. Depression symptoms and mortality in persons aged 65 and over living in the community: a systematic review of the literature. Int J Geriatric Psychiatry. 2001;16:622-30.

[27] Strong K, Mather C, Leeder S, Beaglehole R. Preventing Chronic diseases: How many lives can we save? Lancet. 2005;366:1578-82.

[28] Tatt ID, Barlow KL, Nicoll A. The public health significance of HIV-1 subtypes. AIDS. 2001;15(Suppl 5):S59-71.

[29] Vieweg WV, Julius DA, Fernandez A, et al. Treatmeant of depression in patients with coronary heart disease. Am J Med. 2006;119:567-73.

[30] Wilson D, Naidoo S, Bekker L, Cotton M, Maartens G. Handbook of HIV medicine. Cape Town: Oxford University press; 2002.

[31] Young TN, Arens FJ, Kennedy GE, Laurie JW, Rutherford G. Antiretroviral post-exposure prophylaxis (PEP) for occupational HIV exposure. Cochrane Database Syst Rev. 2007;1(CD002835).

Persistence of HIV-Associated Neurocognitive Disorders in the Era of Antiretroviral Therapy

Jennifer M. King, Brigid K. Jensen,
Patrick J. Gannon and Cagla Akay

Additional information is available at the end of the chapter

1. Introduction

HIV-Associated Neurocognitive Disorders (HAND) is a serious menifestation of HIV infection in the central nervous system (CNS), and encompassess a wide spectrum of cognitive, behavioral, and motor deficits [1-3]. While the implementation of combination antiretroviral therapy (ART) has dramatically increased the life expectancy and led to significant improvements in the clinical presentation and progression of HAND, an estimated 50% of HIV-infected patientscontinue to suffer from implications of HAND in the ART era, with as much as 20% of these exhibiting symptoms of HIV-associated dementia (HAD), the most severe form of HAND [3-6]. The brain regions affected in patients with HAND has changed in the ART era in parallel to the changes observed in the clinical picture; a more subtle and insidious cortical damage mainly in the hippocampus and the temporal cortex is observed, in contrast to the overt subcortical damage seen before ART [7-10]. The underlying causes of these changes are not fully elucidated; however, examination of the post-mortem tissue reveals the persistence of synaptic and dendritic damage in the affected brain regions [3, 11]. Emerging evidence suggests that controlling viral replication in the periphery or in the CNS may not be sufficient to control the underlying neuropathological processes that culminate in the development of HAND. The impact of HAND on the quality of life, adherence to drug regimens, and co-morbidities especially in an aging HIV population with decreased cognitive reserves, is of major concern. In this chapter, we will examine the major factors that continue to impact the CNS of HIV-infected individuals, and introduce new challenges in the successful treatment of HAND.

2. Clinical presentation and neuropathology of HAND

According to the diagnostic criteria established for the assessment of neurocognitive impairment in HIV-infected individuals, the neurological deficits in HAND patients are divided into three diagnostic groups. This classification is based on the neuropsychological evaluation of multiple cognitive domains, including simple motor skills or sensory perceptual ability, complex perceptual motor skills, attention and working memory, learning and memory recall, verbal and language, abstraction and executive function. Asymptomatic neurocognitive impairment (ANI) is defined as acquired impairment in at least two cognitive domains without a decline in activities of daily living (ADL), while mild to moderate neurocognitive impairment that affects ADL is termed minor neurocognitive disorder (MND). Moderate to severe impairment in two or more domains with marked impact on ADL is defined as HAD. Additionally, behavioral and emotional problems such as depression, psychosis and anxiety are commonly observed in HAND patients. Since the multi-drug regimens that form the basis of ART have become the mainstay of HIV, the clinical presentation and the course of HAND have become more unpredictable. The severity of deficits appears to fluctuate over time during the course of infection: some patients may experience continuing decline in cognitive abilities, while others may recover from HAD and exhibit only minor deficits for the remainder of the disease. While clinical studies clearly establish that suppression of viral replication below the level of detection is paramount to a more favorable outcome, the clinical course of HAND, once diagnosed, cannot be predicted successfully in most patients.

While microglial nodules, multinucleated giant cells and astrogliosis, all of which are associated with HIV-induced inflammatory changes, are not as frequently found in post-mortem HAND brain tissue after ART, dendritic and synaptic damage still persist [12-16]. For example, several studies have reported the presence of deoxynucleotidyltransferase-mediated dUTP nick-end labeling (TUNEL)-positive cells, DNA laddering and structural changes with electron microscopy [17, 18]. Importantly, these markers of neuronal death correlate with activation of immune cell populations suggesting that the inflammatory mediators secreted by these cells may play a role in initiating the death cascades [1, 19]. Given the chronic nature of the HIV infection in the ART era, co-existing conditions which can activate immune responses and precipitate a neuroinflammatory environment independent of infection are likely to contribute to the development of persistent neuropathology, and need to be addressed for a more efficient clinical approach and more favorable outcomes. Foremost, it is necessary to examine the mechanisms of neuronal injury in order to successfully expound on the contribution of confounding factors on the persistence of HAND.

The two major cell types targeted by HIV are CD4+ T cells and the cells of monocyte/macrophage lineage. HIV infection of the CD4+ T cells ends in the selective loss of this cell population, leading to severe immunodeficiency [20]. More relevant to HAND, HIV also targets monocytes early during infection [20]. In the healthy brain, the BBB and the blood-cerebrospinal fluid barriers are the first lines of defense against invading pathogens; however, HIV can circumvent these barriers and enter the CNS within infected monocytes [21, 22]. According to this model, supported by a multitude of *in vitro* and *in vivo* studies, the infected monocytes differentiate into macrophages, and constitute the viral reservoirs in the CNS [23-26]. Moreover, these cells release a variety of molecules, some of them known neurotoxins, leading to the eventual neuronal damage and dysfunction observed in HAND. Importantly, unlike other cell types that readily undergo replication, neurons in their post-mitotic state are more vulnerable to immune cell damage which can disrupt critical neuronal functions. Additionally, recent focus in efforts towards a cure in HIV is purging the virus from its reservoirs, by reactivating pro-viral DNA [27-31]. Thus, it is crucial to examine the impact of HIV infection on immune cells for a better understanding of the neuropathology of HAND, and for the development of successful paradigms for HIV reactivation and purging.

3. The immunology of HAND

3.1. Initiation of immune response in the CNS

HIV initially enters helper T lymphocytes and monocytes in the periphery via viral glycoproteins, gp120 and gp41, which are part of the HIV envelope [32]. These glycoproteins engage with the CD4 on the host cell membrane; however, this fusion step requires the presence of a chemokine co-receptor, C-X-C chemokine receptor type 4 (CXCR4) in lymphocytes,orC-C chemokine type 5 (CCR5) / C-C chemokine type 3 (CCR3) in macrophages [32, 33]. Of all the cell types in the brain, only macrophages and microglia express CD4 antigen, are commonly infected by HIV, and are capable of productive infection. There is very limited evidence for HIV infection of the glial cells, which if present, has not been conclusively shown as being productive [34]. More importantly, HIV cannot infect neurons as these cells lack CD4 co-receptors.

The CNS of a healthy adult human has a relatively low presence of cellular components of the immune system [35, 36]. The CNS presents the immune system with unique problems with trafficking of immune cells and the recognition of foreign antigen when present. First, the BBB constitutes a physical barrier for the entry of cells and macromolecules from the periphery into the CNS. Additionally, there is minimal expression of major histocompatibility class II (MHC class II) molecules and an absence of professional antigen presenting cells such as dendritic cells, all of which are required for antigen presentation and adaptive immune response activation. However, it has been extensively shown that brain derived factors act to suppress or counter-regulate the actions of pro-inflammatory mediators in the CNS where immune surveillance is not sufficient. For example, transforming growth factor-β (TGF-β) has the ability to inhibit the activation of macrophages, T lymphocytes, and natural killer (NK) cells, and has been shown to possess neuroprotective capabilities [37-41]. Interestingly, increased TGF-β protein levels are reported in the frontal cortex of HAD patients, and elevated TGF-βimmunoreactivity has been detected in reactive astrocytes and mononuclear cells of the white matter in HIV-infected CNS [42, 43]. Similar roles have been proposed for BDNF, NT-3, and NGF, among others, during HIV infection in the CNS [44, 45].

In the initial stages of HIV infection, the number of CD4+T cells decreases as a consequence of uncontrolled viral replication. While the impact of primary HIV infection on specific CD8+ T cell subpopulations is not clear, there is an overall expansion of this cell population [46]. In this environment, infected monocytes can enter the CNS, establish and maintain productive infection, and HAND becomes clinically manifest. Perivascular macrophages are replenished throughout life by the migration of circulating monocytes to the brain, a process enhanced in an inflammatory environment [47]. Several studies have shown that the number of activated macrophages, rather than the viral load,correlates best with the axonal damage and synaptic loss observed in the HAND brain [11, 14, 48, 49]. In addition, indirect markers of macrophage activation, such as neopterin and β2-microglobulin, are elevated in the CSF of HAND patients [50-52]. Further, soluble factors that are known to be released by macrophages and glia, such as quinolinic acid, tumor necrosis factor-α (TNF-α), reactive oxygen species (ROS), and cytokines such as CXCL12 (stromal cell-derived factor-1, SDF-1), CCL2 (monocyte chemotactic protein-1, MCP-1), and interleukin-6 (IL-6), are also elevated in the CSF of HAND patients [53-57]. These findings reinforce the model which proposes monocyte-derived macrophages and microglia as major instigators of the neuropathological processes in the course of disease development in HAND.

It should be noted that viral proteins such as gp120 and transactivator of transcription (Tat) can directly activate uninfected macrophages [58-62]. Additionally, one mechanism of injury that is proposed to account for neuronal damage in the absence of neuronal infection by HIV involves direct neurotoxicity by these viral proteins. Several *in vitro* studies have shown that these viral proteins that are released and/or shed by the infected macrophages/microglia can induce direct synaptic and neuronal damage [63-65]. However, the indicators of neuroinflammation continue to persist despite successful suppression of replication in the CSF to levels below the limit of detection with ART, suggesting that other, less direct mechanisms of injury might be major contributors to the underlying neuropathology.

3.2. The role of cytokines and chemokines in HAND neuropathology

A number of indirect mechanisms for the pathogenesis of HAND have been proposed [1, 25, 66]. These mechanisms are not mutually exclusive, and may be synergistic based on the common background of macrophage activation and release of cytokines and chemokines.As a protective measure to suppress viral production, macrophages are responsible for the production of inflammatory mediators including TNF-α, IL (interleukin)-1, interferon-α (IFN-α) and nitric oxide synthase (NOS) [33, 59]. However, the release of these pro-inflammatory cytokines can activate the uninfected macrophages, and can induce the migration of leukocytes into the CNS [62]. For example, in HIV-1 transgenic (Tg) rats, elevated levels of IL-1β and TNF-α and increased expression of arachidonic acid cascade enzymes have been implicated in neuronal damage and cognitive and behavioral impairment [67]. A recent study indicates that similar changes could contribute to cognitive impairment in HIV-infected patients despite an effective ART [68]. *In vivo* studies suggest that the progression of HAND may be predicted by high concentrations of TNF-α in plasma, and polymorphisms in the TNF-α promoter are associated with HAND to a degree [69, 70]. Interestingly, functional *ex-*

vivo studies have shown that the macrophages and B-lymphocytes isolated from HIV-infected patients are activated despite viral suppression by ART [71]. Further, *in vitro* experiments show that HIV reactivation can be achieved by cytokine and chemokine stimulation [30, 33]. These findings are especially important in light of recent concerns regarding viral latency and its contribution to the persistence of HAND [29].

In the CNS,chemoattractant cytokines, or chemokines have been demonstrated as essential factors in neuroinflammation and related neuronal injury and loss through their regulation of inflammatory responses. Post-mortem studies have revealed up-regulation of chemokines and chemokine receptors in the brains of patients with HAND [25, 26, 56, 72-75]. The best-characterized chemokines up-regulated in HAND are the β-chemokines CCL2, CCL5, and CX3CL1, and the alpha chemokine CXCL12. For example, the levels of one of the more potent chemokines, CCL2 correlate with the likelihood and severity of HAND [76, 77]. In addition, an intriguing regulatory role for the chemokine CCR5 was demonstrated that its activation led to cell death via caspase-3 mediated apoptosis in a neuroblastoma cell line [78]. Further, induction of apoptosis has also been reported with CXCL12 in primary neuroglial cultures in the absence of the HIV viral protein gp120. However, results from several recent studies suggest that the changes in the expression of these chemokines may indicate neuroprotective efforts in response to the neuroinflammatory environment [79]. Further studies are needed to dissect the roles of chemokines in HAND pathogenesis, as they take part in a crucial phase in immune responses, and provide attractive targets for modulation in resolving HAND persistence.

The mechanisms by which the neuroinflammatory environment eventually ends in damage to the neurons are not precisely known; however, several mechanisms are likely candidates. Studies suggest that the neuronal damageis a result of indirect effects of viral proteins as well as inflammatory mediators [1, 66]. Gp120 and Tat are reported to induce neuronal apoptosis by activating death-associated proteases, caspases, specifically caspase-3 in *in vitro* and *in vivo* disease models [80]. Another mechanism proposes a role for excitotoxicity secondary to impaired glutamate reuptake by astrocytes which are overwhelmed by pro-inflammatory factors [81]. The well-defined cascade of excitotoxic injury includes excess Ca^{2+} influx into the neuronal cytoplasm. Several downstream events secondary to such increases in Ca^{2+} such as excess free radical production and oxidative stress, and the activation of Ca^{2+}-dependent death proteases, calpains and caspases, will be detrimental to neurons, especially in an environment with inadequate glial support and ongoing inflammation due to immune cell activation [1, 66].

3.3. Neuroinflammation in HAND

The persistence of immune activation in the CNS and the peripheral nervous system (PNS) of HIV-infected individuals in the ART era is supported by several lines of evidence. The relatively low levels of HIV RNA in the presence of widespread neuropathological changes in the CNS and PNS of HAND patients, and the lack of evidence of HIV infection of neuronal cells *in vivo and in vitro* hint at the possibility of chronic immune activation as a factor in the persistence of HAND. Recent clinical evidence shows that ART reduces intrathecal immunoactivation in treated patients; however, a significant percentage of patients continue to exhibit signs of ongoing inflammation [49, 50, 82, 83]. Further, even after successful reduction of HIV RNA levels below the limit of detection for several years, patients present with increased levels of inflammatory markers such as CSF neopterin and intrathecal IgG [52]. It is thus apparent that ART is not sufficient to prevent or control HAND. One major factor to consider in addressing this failure is that ART may not be efficient and/or sufficient in controlling the inflammatory cascade triggered by HIV infection.

Once HIV replication is established in the CNS, the initial chemotactic and inflammatory factor production leads to further recruitment and activation of monocytes/macrophages, creating a perpetual neuroinflammatory environment. The phenomenon of monocyte/macrophage recruitment can be explained by a "push and pull" mechanism [47]. Two key chemokines that play a role in the recruitment, or "pull", of monocytes are CCL2 and fractalkine (CXCL1).CCL2 is considered to be the more critical factor involved in the infiltration of monocytes and lymphocytes across the BBB in the HAND brain [79]. Multiple cell types of the CNS have been shown to produce CCL2 in models of inflammation, in which CCL2 is a part of a signaling mechanism for recruitment of monocytes/macrophages from the periphery. For example, leukocyte infiltration into the brain parenchyma has been demonstrated upon pertussis toxin challenge in CCL2 transgenic mice [84]. More importantly, HIV-infected leukocyte transmigration across BBB is dependent on CCL2 in an *in vitro* model of disease [85]. Further, CCL2 has been shown to directly damage the endothelial cell junctions of the BBB [86]. These findings clearly indicate a significant role for CCL2 in the "pull" of monocyte/macrophages across the BBB in HAND. Interestingly, CCL2 levels remain elevated in the CSF of HAND patients on ART, implicating that ongoing trafficking might be occurring despite viral suppression, and warrants further investigations into the persistence of HAND in the era of ART [83].

The "push" aspect of the monocyte/macrophage recruitment involves the expansion in peripheral blood neuroinvasive monocyte population. It has been shown that individuals with HAND exhibit an expanded population of CD14+ peripheral blood monocytes that co-express CD16, which is considered a more mature population [21]. These CD14+/CD16+ monocytes are preferentially susceptible to infection, and can serve as a reservoir harboring proviral DNA. The entry of monocytes into the brain plays a key role in initiating the series of events that lead to HAND, and although antiretrovirals hinder viral replication, they may have minimal effects on the continued transmigration of monocytes into the brain. One study showed that a single exposure of the CNS to the neurotoxic viral protein Tat led to the infiltration of peripheral blood monocytes and resulted in prolonged disruption of CNS function [87]. Thus, continuous and efficient viral suppression in the periphery is critical in achieving suppressed inflammation in the CNS, and is of prime importance in the fight against HAND.

While macrophages and microglia play primary roles in HIV infection in the CNS, other glial cells also contribute to the neuroinflammation and neurotoxicity in the HAND brain. One important cell type that needs to be mentioned in the neuroinflamatory processes in HAND is the astrocytic cell population. As the most abundant cells in the CNS, astrocytes provide neurotrophic support, and are involved in repair processes for neurons. Further, astrocytes are physiological regulators of microglial and macrophage inflammatory responses, and indirectly modulate neuronal survival through reduction of the macrophage inflammatory response. However, their dysfunction, as a result of HIV infection, will lead to the dysregulation of the local cytokine/chemokine balance. Evidence has shown that astrocytes are key mediators in the regulation of microglial function and its influence on the onset and the progression of HAND [55, 88]. Viral proteins gp120, and Tat both activate astrocytes to produce pro-inflammatory cytokines TNF-α, IL-6, and IL-1β as well as the pro-inflammatory chemokines CCL2 and CXCL10 [34, 55, 89-91]. The contribution of these pro-inflammatory mediators by astrocytes as well as the release of pro-inflammatory cytokines IL-1β and TNF-α by microglia and macrophage will only exacerbate the inflammatory environment in the HIV-infected CNS.

Although the pathogenic mechanisms of HAND are likely to be multifactorial (Table 1), cellular activation with the initiation and persistence of the immune system in the CNS play a pivotal role in this disease progression. Continued CNS inflammation is an essential factor in many neurodegenerative diseases and HIV infection induces a cascade of inappropriate immune responses in the CNS. The initial immunological response has protective intentions through macrophage activation, but with persistent infection, the inflammatory response becomes toxic to the neurons through the production of pro-inflammatory cytokines and chemokines. Further, the decreased viral load in the CNS is accompanied by persistent microglial activation and inflammation. Ineffective drug penetrance into the CNS, which continues to be a challenge, can initiate the development of resistance to ART via permitting mutations to the virus which allows the CNS to become a reservoir for the infection. As HIV-infected macrophages are shown to be resistant to apoptosis, this will end in exacerbating the virus reservoir in the CNS.

Inflammatory Responses During HIV-1 Brain Infection
Macrophage Activation (M1 phenotype)
Micogial nodules
Multinucleated Giant Cells in Central White Matter and Deep Gray Matter
Astrogliosis
Cytokines
Transforming Growth Factor-beta (TGF-β)
Tumor Necrosis Factor-alpha(TNF-α)
Interleukin-6 (IL-6)
Interleukin-1 (IL-1)
Chemokines
Monocyte Chemotactic Protein-1 (MCP-1)
Interferon Gamma Induced Protein-10 (IP-10)
MHC class II presentation

Table 1. Pathological and laboratory evidence for immune activation in the CNS after HIV infection.

It should also be noted that the impact of HIV infection in the peripheral tissue will ultimately impact the immune responses in the CNS. Thus, co-morbidities such as co-infections,
substance abuse, malignancies and antiretroviral drug toxicities, as well as general inflammatory processes in the periphery, such as oxidative stress should be taken into account
when assessing the relationships between immune responses and the neuropathological
processes occurring in the HAND brain. This approach will provide more efficient tools,
and will have a greater impact on resolving the persistence of HAND.

4. Oxidative stress in neurodegenerative diseases

Oxidative stress is a shared pathological finding in a myriad of neurodegenerative diseases
including Alzheimer Disease, Parkinson Disease, Multiple Sclerosis (MS), Amyotrophic Lateral Sclerosis (ALS), and HAND [92, 93]. While it is clear that chronic oxidative stress which
will overwhelm the protective capacities of the cellular endogenous antioxidant responses
may be responsible in part for the neuronal death occurring in these conditions, in many
neurodegenerative diseases it is difficult to ascertain whether oxidative stress is the causative factor for disease pathology and progression, or rather a resultant downstream event of
other cellular dysfunctions [92-95]. Nonetheless, in HAND, several lines of evidence suggest
that both HIV and antiretroviral compounds may result in oxidative and nitrosative stress in
the periphery and in the CNS [96-102]. Deficits in total antioxidant levels and increases in
the markers for oxidative stress are still observed in individuals on stable ART regimens
with undetectable viral titers, necessitating the need for adjunctive therapies to ameliorate
this imbalance [103, 104]. As has been suggested in a variety of neurodegenerative conditions, antioxidant supplementation or upregulation of the endogenous antioxidant response
in cells of the CNS may ameliorate the neuronal damage and death in HAND [1, 93, 94, 105].

4.1. Oxidative stress in the era of ART

The evidence of disrupted antioxidant balance and oxidative stress represent a continued
concern for HIV-infected individuals even when virus is successfully controlled by ART
[102]. To understand the magnitude and implications of this problem, it is important to understand the initial disruptions to the antioxidant system that were observed in infected individuals, and determine whether ART contributed to the resolution or the exacerbation of
these problems.

Oxidative stress prior to ART:As early as 1988, while researchers were just beginning to understand the HIV virus, Sönnerborg and colleagues determined that plasma levels of malondialdehyde in adults with HIV infection were elevated up to 30% when compared with
controls [106]. Malondialdehyde is the breakdown product of polyunsaturated lipids by reactive oxygen species, and is a mainstay in terms of a biological marker for measuring the
relative levels of lipid peroxidation and oxidative stress in individuals [107]. A multitude of
studies followed, showing significant increases in the levels of free radicals, hydroperoxides,
hydroxynoneal, and oxidation of thiols in infected individuals, and confirming that malon-

dialdehyde is increased significantly in infected adults, as well as children [108-118]. The metabolic synthesis of lipids is closely tied to the oxidative state of the cell and the lipids residing in the cell membrane, as certain enzymes such as sphingomyelinase, are sensitive to the oxidative status of the cell and regulate their activity based on cellular need [119]. Studies looking into the production of sphingolipids illustrated an overproduction of both sphingomyelin and ceramides with HIV-infection, suggesting a lipid imbalance caused by the virus [115, 116, 119]. Additionally, studies showed remarkable deficiencies in antioxidant micronutrients including zinc, selenium, Vitamin C, Vitamin D, Vitamin E and beta-carotene (Vitamin A) [109, 110, 118, 120-126]. Conflicting reports exist on perturbation of total antioxidant status prior to ART, with severalclinical studies reporting decreased total antioxidant capacity [108, 113, 118], while Repetto et al. described an increase in the overall antioxidant capacity as individuals progressed to AIDS [114]. The discrepancies between these findings are likely based on the assays utilized to determine "total antioxidant capacity", as different enzymatic approaches target different portions of the antioxidant system.

Activity levels of superoxide dismutase (SOD), which catalyzes the detoxification of the oxidant superoxide into hydrogen peroxide and water, were assessed by a variety of laboratories. Elevated SOD activity was observed in all evaluated HIV-infected individuals, with further increases occuringwith disease progression to AIDS. In addition, increases in SOD mRNA levels were reported in individuals with HAD, as compared to those who were neurocognitively normal [114, 127, 128]. These changes in SOD were observed in microglial cells, as well as in HIV-infected macrophages, suggesting a virus-triggered induction [128]. An essential antioxidant found in the brain which buffers many reactive oxygen species is glutathione. In HIV-infected patients, overall glutathione levels were found to be reduced, and the remaining glutathione was greatly skewed to the oxidized versus reduced form. [114, 127, 129, 130]. The enzyme glutathione peroxidase, which promotes the conversion of hydrogen peroxide to water through the use of glutathione, was also decreased, illustrating a severe imbalance in this system whose goal is to maintain cellular redox homeostasis [121]. Another deleterioius consequence of rampant pro-oxidants within cells is oxidative modification of DNA bases. Increased levels of 5-hydroxyuracil, 5-hydroxycytosine, 8-hydroxyadenine and 8-hydroxyguanine were found when comparing DNA isolated from lymphocytes of HIV-infected individuals versus uninfected controls [131]. One other common product of an imbalanced oxidative state which is beginning to gain more interest and research focus is peroxynitrite. This compound, which is formed when superoxide reacts with nitric oxide, is detectable through its nitrotyrosine moiety, and is found at higher levels and with more frequency in the brains of patients with HAD, compared with those who are neurocognitively normal [128]. In addition to the generation of superoxide as a direct result of HIV infection, the virus also increases mRNA expression of inducible nitric oxide synthase (iNOS), which enables a precipitous accumulation of this deleterious oxidation product [128].Further research in the Nath laboratory has illustrated that thirteen proteins with nitrotyrosine modifications are present in the CSF of individuals with HIV-infection. Individuals with dementia had the highest levels of these nitrites and nitrates. Importantly, three of these proteins were significantly elevated in individuals who showed declines in neurocognitive assessment over a period of 6 months [101].

While it appears that there is not an all-or-nothing increase or decrease in antioxidant capacity, the evidence is clear that the components of the antioxidant defense system prior to ART were greatly affected by HIV-infection, and that the capabilities of endogenous antioxidant response were not able to alleviate damaging oxidative alterations to proteins and DNA.

Persistence of oxidative stress in the era of ART: In the ART era, oxidative stress is still pervasive in individuals living with well controlled HIV-infection [102]. In 2007, a group at the University of Pennsylvania sought to ascertain whether ART had an effect on inflammation and oxidative stress in the brains of HIV-infected individuals through utilization of chemical-shift magnetic resonance spectroscopy. Through careful analysis of lipid, lactate, and creatine levels, they determined that the inflammation and oxidative stress initiated by the HIV infection was not ameliorated in ART-treated individuals, compared to seronegative controls [132]. While these effects were observed in all HAND patients, the levels of oxidative stress markers were higher in those with more severe cognitive deficits [132].

Lipid peroxidation is still rampant despite effective viral control. While a couple of studies report decreased levels in markers of lipid peroxidation in ART-medicated patients, as compared with those not receiving ART, multiple studies have shown persistent statistically significant increases in hydroperoxides, isoprostanes, and malondialdehyde in ART-treated HIV-infected individuals, compared to seronegative controls [103, 113, 133-139]. Interestingly, two independent groups have determined in patient blood samples that the levels of peroxide species and oxidative stress are higher in patients on protease inhibitor (PI) based regimens, as compared with those in individuals on non-nucleoside reverse transcriptase inhibitor (NNRTI) based regimens, implicating a role for the protease inhibitor class in induction or exacerbation of oxidative stress [138, 140].

Micronutrient deficiencies are still problematic with ART, and while most patients have adequate plasma concentrations of vitamins C, D, and E, reported levels are still considered sub-optimal and lower than seronegative patients [123, 141]. While subsequent reports have indicated that zinc and selenium deficits are no longer observed in individuals on ART, further definitive confirmation of these findings is necessary [142, 143]. Additionally, in studies which evaluated the serum of adults and the saliva of children, the total antioxidant status was found to be decreased in ART treated HIV-patients when compared to HIV-negative controls, mirroring findings in studies conducted in the pre-ART era [104, 144].

While several studies have indicated that introduction of ART has been accompanied by an improvement in overall glutathione status, this effect is not totally rectified and imbalances still occur [129]. In particular, numerous groups have shown that circulating glutathione levels are still markedly reduced in HIV-infected individuals, when compared with age-matched controls, with the ratio of oxidized to reduced glutathione remaining out of balance [112, 133-135, 145]. Unfortunately, studies investigating nitrosative stress and nitrosylated proteins in HIV-infected individuals on ART are still lacking; however, the Nath, Hammond, and Sutliff laboratories have been investigating nitrosative stress in HIV, and it is likely that such reports are forthcoming.

It has been reported that HIV-positive individuals do not have altered levels of 8-hydroxy-2'-deoxyguanosine [8-oxoG) in their urine regardless of ART or lipodystrophy status [146]. While these findings appear to be promising, in a very recent study, autopsy tissue from frontal cortex was stained for both nuclear and mitochondrial 8-oxoG. The levels of this oxidized DNA product were significantly increased in cases of HAND, suggesting that ART, or ART in combination with ongoing infection may promote DNA oxidative modification, cellular dysfunction damage and death [147]. Additionally, the presence of clastogenic factors, which cause chromosomal breaks and DNA damage and which may be released from cells under conditions of oxidative stress, was observed in the plasma of all HIV-patients tested by Edeas *et al.* [148]. This was true of patients that were both asymptomatic and symptomatic for AIDS-defining pathologies, and was independent of ART status [148]. The effects of these clastogenic factors appear to persist in multiple cell populations implicated in HAND pathogenesis. For example, in leukocytes obtained from HIV-infected individuals, the percentage of cells exhibiting DNA fragmentation was increased in individuals on ART, as compared with those who were ART- naïve [135]. However, the results of this study have not addressed the possible contribution of latent or low level of infection to the findings. Due to pervasive oxidative damage and antioxidant imbalance despite effective long-term viral control in patients, it is now imperative to recognize the direct effect that viral enclaves and antiretroviral drugs themselves may have on perpetuating these effects. Further studies are needed to investigate the independent effects of ART and the virus on oxidative damage in the CNS, as well as in the periphery in order to better determine therapeutic interventions to resolve these dysfunctions.

4.2. Oxidative stress induction by HIV

Exhaustive research has been conducted in order to determine the effects of the HIV on infected cells and the cytotoxic factors released from these cells. As addressed earlier, it is now clear that HIV-infected macrophages secrete a variety of neurotoxic substances including glutamate, nitric oxide, and superoxide [96]. Within actively infected human myeloid-monocytic cell lines or monocyte-derived macrophages, HIV induces an increase in superoxide anions, with a concomitant increase in superoxide to combat these factors [128, 149]. Mollace and colleagues have demonstrated that the supernatants from HIV-infected human primary macrophages induced oxidative stress in astrocytes, as indicated by increases in malondialdeyde levels [150]. They further showed that these supernatants, which contained excess superoxide, induced astrocytic apoptosis, confirming HIV-mediated toxicity of this secreted product [150]. In a similar fashion, in HIV-infected monocytes, an induction of nitric oxide synthase and subsequent increase nitric oxide was observed [151]. It is also interesting to note that elevated oxidative stress in the form of intracellular singlet oxygen is capable of reactivating latent HIV through long terminal repeat (LTR) transactivation in infected monocytes or lymphocytes, suggesting that the virus may rely on oxidative stress signaling cascades for continuation of long-term infection or viral rebound [152].

The amino acid and neurotransmitter glutamate is normally secreted from neurons into the synaptic cleft, and is quickly removed and recycled through the actions of astrocytes. This molecule normally activates the N-methyl D-aspartate (NMDA) receptor on neurons, and allows for Ca^{2+} entry into the cell. However, it has been clearly demonstrated that excessive extracellular levels of glutamate resulting from overstimulation of neurons, impaired reuptake by astrocytes, or release from other cell populations within the brain can lead to hyperactivation of NMDA channels, subsequent increases in Ca^{2+} levels in the neuronal cytoplasm, resulting in excitotoxic neuronal death [153]. In 2001, Jiang et al. demonstrated through a series of elegant experiments that the molecule responsible for the neurotoxicity observed on neuronal cultures was a molecule of less than 3,000 kilodaltons, was not sensitive to trypsin digestion, and that its neurotoxic effect was blocked by a selective NMDA receptor antagonist, MK-801. It was through this study, as well as a subsequent study by O'Donnell et al. that the increased levels of extracellular glutamate secreted by HIV-infected macrophages may be a major factor in HIV-infected macrophage mediated indirect neuronal death [154]. The increases in extracellular glutamate appears to be an effect of dysregulation of the glutamate synthesis pathway, as inhibition of the mitochondrial glutaminase enzyme blocks the production and the secretion of glutamate from HIV-infected macrophages [155-157]. As was distinctly noted in human patient samples, a marked deficiency of glutathione and an imbalance between the oxidized and the reduced glutathione was observed. Within cells, glutaminase is the enzyme which converts glutamine to glutamate. It is tempting to consider that the oxidative stress resulting from the lack of the antioxidant properties of glutamine may be very tightly coupled to a depletion of glutamine from cells by hyperactivation of glutaminase enzymes, precipitating an overproduction of glutamate and triggering an excitotoxic neuronal death pathway.

Similar to effects of whole virus *in vivo*, when gp120 and Tat were injected into the brains of rats, both of these viral proteins induced lipid peroxidation and glutathione depletion [158]. Additionally, both of these proteins significantly reduced intracellular glutathione, and increased malondialdehyde in immortalized brain endothelial cells, showing that the oxidative status of these cells would also be directly affected by the presence of virus. This is of particular importance as the altered oxidative status of these endothelial cells comprising the BBB will have potential impact on not only the integrity of the BBB, but also on the monocyte/macrophage transmigration to the CNS, an important factor in the persistence of HAND [159]. Further, when applied to neurons in culture, gp120 and Tat induce disruptions in the lipid metabolism, leading to increased levels of sphingomyelin, ceramide, and hydroxynoneal,paralleling disruptions in these pathways observed in the neurons of HAND patients [116].

Studies that investigated gp120 separately have revealed that it is capable of inducing ROS formation, and activating the antioxidant response in astrocytes [91, 160]. Studies looking into the production of oxidant species by gp120 have shown that superoxide ions as well as nitric oxide are involved in neuronal toxicity [100, 161]. Mechanistically, gp120-induced nitric oxide formation is dependent on a mannose-specific endocytic lectin in macrophages, while gp120-induced expression and upregulation of iNOS selectively occurs in astrocytes in human fetal neuroglial cultures [100, 162]. Multiple studies have shown that in neurons undergoing gp120-induced toxicity, a significant increase in intracellular Ca^{2+}, likely released from intracellular stores, preceeded death, suggesting at a mechanism of activation of calpains or other pro-death cellular machinery [63, 160].

Studies investigating Tat-induced neuronal death have revealed that this viral protein triggered the accumulation of ROS when exogenously applied to a variety of cell types, including lymphocytes, microglia, brain microvascular endothelial cells (BMECs) and neurons, as well as in HeLa cells expressing Tat [163-166]. When directly injected into striatum of rats, Tat produced dramatic increases in protein oxidative modifications and protein carbonyls [167]. Protein carbonyls were also markedly increased in HeLa cells expressing Tat, supporting *in vivo* data [166]. In addition, decreased levels of glutathione were observed in cardiac myocytes and BMECs exposed to recombinant Tat protein, Tat-expressing transgenic mice, and in Tat-expressing HeLa cells [164, 168-170]. Two studies pinpointed the involvement of manganese-dependent superoxide dismutase (Mn-SOD) as a key player in Tat- induced cellular changes. By expressing Tat in HeLa cells, the laboratories of Lehman and McCord convincingly showed that Tat suppressed the RNA, protein, and activity levels of Mn-SOD, while inducing no changes in the Cu,Zn SOD enzyme levels [166, 170]. In HIV-infected individuals, plasma levels of SOD were increased in plasma, and these changes were in parallel with disease progression to AIDS. If the results from these HeLa cell studies can be expanded to other cell populations, it is tempting to speculate that perhaps this overall increase in SOD activity is a compensatory mechanism resulting from the Tat-induced alterations in Mn-SOD activity and the subsequent increases in superoxide ions that cannot be eliminated. The overexpression of Tat in HeLa cells also led to decreases in overall glutathione levels, with a lower ratio of reduced to oxidized glutathione in the remaining supply, mimicking the effect seen in HIV-infected individuals *in vivo* and in HIV-infected macrophages *in vitro* [166, 170].

Finally, studies focusing on microglia have shown that the expression of HIV viral protein R (Vpr) can induce oxidative stress pathways, and can activate HIV latent gene expression [171]. When exogenously applied to human fetal astrocytes, the oxidative stress caused by Vpr causes decreases in intracellular ATP and glutathione, and skews remaining glutathione in favor of the oxidized versus reduced form [172].

In summary, exhaustive *in vivo* and *in vitro* studies indicate that HIV viral proteins themselves can induce, precipitate and augment oxidative stress in multiple cell types, of both peripheral and CNS tissue. These findings further emphasize the importance of complete inhibition of viral replication in alleviating oxidative stress via antiretroviral therapy. However, emerging evidence suggests that antiretroviral drugs themselves might inadvertently lead to oxidative stress.

4.3. Oxidative stress and ART

Due to the requirement for lifelong adherence to antiretroviral regimens to prevent viremia and immune system compromise, it is necessary to investigate the effects of these compounds in a cellular context. Many of these drugs are associated with negative side effects, and have been linked to the metabolic syndrome, atherosclerosis, lipodystrophy, proteasome inhibition and the unfolded protein response [173-175]. Additionally, it has become apparent that these compounds themselves produce oxidative stress, even in the absence of virus, and may in fact be contributing to the persistence of oxidative stress in patients with well controlled viral load [97, 102].

HIV is highly susceptible to mutations, mostly due to the error-prone reverse transcription step during replication, and underlies the emergence of drug resistant mutations over time in patients treated with single antiretroviral drugs in the early 1990s. Additionally, the development of more sensitive methods for HIV RNA detection revealed the presence of viral reservoirs in multiple tissues, including the CNS. These findings led to the revision of antiretroviral therapy, which, until that time included mostly single antiretroviral drug regimens. A multiple drug treatment approach, termed ART, was implemented to aim at different steps in the HIV replication. Currently recommended ART regimens include a cocktail of nucleoside/nucleotide reverse-transcriptaseinhibitors (NRTIs/NtRTIs), non-nucleoside reverse-transcriptase inhibitors (nNRTIs), protease inhibitors (PIs), and to a lesser extent, entry inhibitors and integrase inhibitors(Panel on Antiretroviral Guidelines for Adults and Adolescents. Guidelines for the use of antiretroviral agents in HIV-1-infected adults and adolescents.Department of Health and Human Services.Available at http://aidsinfo.nih.gov/contentfiles/lvguidelines/AdultandAdolescentGL.pdf). This approach has led to improved immune function, long-term viral suppression; and underlies the reductions in HIV-associated morbidity and mortality in the era of ART. The recently updated guidelines recommend ART initiation to all HIV- infected, ART-naive individuals irrespective of CD4$^+$ counts and the impact of early initiation of ART on HIV-associated neurological complications remain to be seen. While a concensus has been reached regarding the time to initiate ART based on CD4 cell counts, AIDS-defining illnesses, and certain co-morbidity factors; the panel did not clearly outline strategies to best eradicate the viral reservoirs in the CNS, and to decrease the risk of developing HAND among infected patients.

In the meantime, one major approach to better control HAND has been to implement therapies that include drugs which achieve therapeutic concentrations in the CNS. While HIV can circumvent the BBB barrier, complex drug transport and efflux mechanisms at this junction hampers effective antiretroviral concentrations in the brain parenchyma. Recent efforts to address this hurdle have led to the establishment of CNS penetrance effectiveness (CPE) score, an algorithm based on the chemical structure, pharmacodynamic and pharmacokinetic data of antiretroviral drugs [176-178]. In summary, an antiretroviral drug with high CPE score is small in size (molecular mass below 400-500 kDa), has high lipid solubility and low protein binding, and it is not a substrate for drug transport or efflux proteins. Unfortunately, results of several clinical studies which incorporated CPE into the design and the analysis of outcomes are not conclusive [176, 178-183]. While a positive correlation between CPE scores and neurological outcomes are observed in several studies, one study revealed that ART regimens with higher CPE scores might be associated with worse neurocognitive performance [184].

These studies investigating the effect of CPE scores on neurological outcomes have inherent caveats. First, due to the limited methodologies, the clinical studies cannot assess the drug concentrations in the brain parenchyma, and instead depend on the CSF levels, which are usually based on measurements after a single-dose administration of the drug. Several factors, such as poor drug adherence and the impact of co-prescribed drugs on the pharmacokinetics of antiretroviral drugs can impact the CNS concentrations and can confound the measured outcomes.additionally, the escape of drug-resistant viral species into the CNS and their establishment in viral reservoirs early during infection can lead to the rise of drug-resistant HIV species in the CNS, and can hinder the efforts to assess the impact of CPE scores on neurological outcomes. Further, co-morbidity factors impacting the integrity of the BBB should also be considered in assessing drug availability in the CNS. Among these factors are cancer, infections, and drug and alcohol abuse, all of which are shown to alter BBB integrity independent of HIV infection, and should be considered when CPE scores are established and evaluated [185-187]. One final factor to consider in evaluating the long-term effectiveness of ART is the potential direct toxicities of antiretroviral drugs in the CNS, especially given the interest in implementation of ART regimens with better CNS penetrance and possibly developing nanoART as part of treatment plans. Antiretroviral drugs have known side-effects in the periphery, including dyslipidemia, and lipohypertrophy. Further, antiretroviral drug-associated toxicity is well documented in the peripheral nervous system, and potential CNS toxicities secondary to ART exist. Oxidative damage elicited by antiretroviral drugs is of particular interest, given ample evidence of ongoing oxidative stress in the HAND brain, as described above.

In several cavalier studies, researchers eloquently demonstrated in several cell populations (human adipocytes, monocytes, myeloid cell lines, and human aortic endothelial cells) that a variety of drugs from the PI and NRTI families, alone or in combinations, induced the production of ROS, hydrogen peroxide, and factors promoting monocyte recruitment. The compounds reported to induce these changes included PIs: indinavir, nelfinavir, lopinavir, ritonavir, saquinavir, atazanavir and NRTIs: stavudine (d4T), zidovudine (AZT), and didanosine [97-99, 188-191]. The compounds amprenavir (PI) and abacavir (NRTI) were consistently reported as lacking these effects, making these drugs good candidates for inclusion in regimens to be prescribed to patients with HAND [98].

As the first available antiretroviral drug, AZT has been extensively studied. While AZT may not be a mainstay drug of choice for customized optimal regimens, as the primary ART compound available in resource-limited developing countries, it is still of importance to understand its cellular effects. AZT was approved for treatment in 1987, and as early as 1992 the Papoian laboratory reported deficits in mitochondrial enzymes and uncoupling of the electron transport chain (ETC) [192]. The disruption of the ETC is a primary cause of mitochondrial based intracellular ROS accumulation and mitochondrial DNA oxidation, an effect since expounded upon in multiple laboratories after acute AZT exposure in isolated heart mitochondria and primary human cardiomyocytes, and after chronic gestational AZT exposure in mouse liver and kidney and in the lung and brain of fetal patas monkeys [193-196]. This compound has also been shown to increase mitochondrial lipid peroxidation, deplete intracellular glutathione, and lead to oxidation of remaining glutathione, ultimately inducing a caspase-3- and caspase-7- dependent apoptotic death [193, 195, 197]. When another NRTI, d4T was investigated, it also was shown to produce ROS, mitochondrial oxidative stress, oxidized mitochondrial DNA, and altered activity of mitochondrial oxidative phosphorylation enzymes [198, 199]. Similarly, NRTI zalcitabine (ddC) also induces oxidative stress, as evidenced by the accumulation of protein carbonyls and nitrotyrosine modifications. Interestingly, this study also reported that the better-tolerated cytidine analog lamivudine (3TC) did not produce these effects, suggesting that 3TC may be considered as an alternative to reduce oxidative stress, and that future compounds generated from this structural base may behave similarly [200]. Interestingly, in contrast to studies in human lymphoid cells, Brandmann and collegues have recently reported that in astrocytes AZT, lamivudine, efavirenz, and nevirapine do not appear to reduce intracellular levels of glutathione [190]. Whether or not these compounds behave similarly in neurons and other cell populations in the CNS remains to be elucidated.

In the non-nucleoside reverse transcriptase inhibitor (nNRTI) drug class, efavirenz applied to a human hepatoblastoma cell line resulted in superoxide generation, depletion of intracellular glutathione, and decrease in mitochondrial function and membrane potential that was independent of mitochondrial DNA replication [201]. In addition, efavirenz has also been linked to neuropsychological side effects in HIV-infected patients, and it is probable that the specific oxidative stress effects on mitochondria and glutathione may play a role in the neurotoxicity of this compound, as neurons are particularly sensitive to perturbations in the antioxidant system [201, 202].

Within the protease inhibitor class, both ritonavir and amprenavir have been associated with increased superoxide anion production, while ritonavir has been shown to cause increases in nitrotyrosine levels in porcine coronary arteries [203]. On the other hand, both indinavir and nelfinavir have been shown to induce a time and concentration dependent depletion of intracellular glutathione in astrocytes as well as in pancreatic beta cells [99, 190]. Nelfinavir is of particular interest, as it suppresses cytosolic, rather than mitochondrial superoxide dismutase levels, and induces a necrotic rather than apoptotic cell death cascade in an adipocyte cell line [99, 204]. Future studies of this compound will undoubtedly prove interesting and may have important implications in patients with regard to their neurocognitive outcomes associated with this compund. Finally, it is interesting to note that multiple studies investigating the oxidative effects of the thymidine analogs in the NRTI class have reported increased ROS, hydrogen peroxide, and nitric oxide intermediates but no superoxide anions [188, 205].

Currently, there is no information on possible oxidative effects of the entry inhibitor, integrase inhibitor, and mutation inhibitor drug classes. Similarly, the lack of published studies for the neuroglial cell populations in the brains of HAND patients is surprising. Several posters at national and international meetings over recent years have addressed this important issue, and hopefully these reports will be forthcoming [206, 207]. In order to design custom drug regimens which will not precipitate, or can ameloirate oxidative stress, cellular dysfunction and death, it is critical to have an understanding of the cellular effects of each currently approved antiretroviral compound, and to design future compounds with minimal oxidative effects. Further, it is possible that the continued dysfunction in superoxide production and superoxide dismutase levels in patients may be due to the effects of more than one drug in a multi-drug regimen. Thus, designing future combinations which do not precipiateoxidative stressis of utmost importance in efforts to resolve the persistence of HAND observed in the ART era.

4.4. Potential therapeutic avenues for oxidative stress in ART era

Since the manifestations of oxidative stress induced by HIV and ART have emerged, it has also become evident to scientists that boosting the endogenous antioxidant response may be a valid and encouraging adjunctive therapeutic option. Within the cell, the antioxidant response is mediated through the activation of transcription factor NF-E2 (nuclear factor (erythroid-derived 2)-related factor-2 (Nrf2)and its myriad of effector phase II and III detoxifying enzymes. Relevant to the previously discussed aberrations in oxidant detoxification, this pathway upregulates superoxide dismutase, peroxiredoxins, thioredoxins, and multiple glutathione biosynthesis enzymes [208, 209].

In vitro, multiple compounds which act upon the Nrf2 pathway have proven effective in ameliorating the oxidative effects of viral infection, viral proteins or antiretroviral drugs. Among these compounds are resveratrol, dimethyl fumarate, N-acetylcysteine, and curcurmin [189, 191, 193, 203, 210]. Antioxidants which have not yet been shown to act through the Nrf2 pathway, but which have similar effects *in vitro* include dihydroxybenzyl alcohol, water soluble vitamin E (trolox), glutathione mimetic tricyclodecan-9-yl-xanthogenat, and acetyl-l-carnitine [188, 200, 201, 211]. An alternative approach to specifically inhibit the actions of NADPH oxidase through the compound diphenyleneiodonium, was able to specifically prevent the effects of PIs, but not NRTIs in human adipocytes [98]. This interesting finding suggests that the different antiretroviral classes may lead to ROS production through different mechanisms, and that specific therapeutics targeting individual oxidant-producing enzymes or pathways may need to be considered for specific ART regimens.

An alternative approach to activating Nrf2 pathway is supplementation with the antioxidant vitamin C (ascorbate), which is capable of directly scavenging reactive oxygen and nitrogen species. This method has been shown to be effective in counteracting the deleterious effects of gp120, as well as nelfinavir *in vitro*, and has been shown to have beneficial outcomes in patients, when supplemented to ART regimens [100, 195, 204]. Along these same lines, supplementation with a variety of other antioxidants and micronutrients including minocycline, glutathione replenishing peptide alpha-lipoic acid, selenium, vitamin A, Vitamin E, and a multivitamin regimen including vitamins A, C, E selenium and coenzyme Q10 have demonstrated partial protection from the deleterious oxidative effects of HIV/SIV and ART *in vivo*, with particular emphasis on restoration of the total blood glutathione levels [127, 195, 212-214]. Finally, the NMDA-receptor blocker memantine, and monoamide oxidase type B inhibitor selegiline, approved for treatment in Alzheimer and Parkinson Diseases, respectively, have also been proposed as potential therapeutics for HAND [1, 214]. Memantine might exert therapeutic effects through reduction of residual virus-mediated glutamate excitotoxicity, and selegiline has been reported to be capable of reducing oxygen-based free radicals [215, 216]. The use of these compounds and their efficacy in reducing oxidative damage in HAND are still in early stages. Initial studies were confounded by the fact that much damage was already present in late stage HAD patients and a protective effect at this stage was not evident [217]. Further work with these compounds will require identifying patients with ANI or MND to enroll in longitudinal studies to determine whether these compounds will have long-term benefit.

Going forward, it is imperative that the oxidative stress imposed by HIV and ART are targeted by adjunctive therapies. As research progresses with the quest for eliminating viral reservoirs and designing more effective, less toxic antiretroviral compounds, it is important to keep in mind that oxidative stress is and will continue to be a persistent burden, especially in a patient population with a significantly enhanced life expectancy.

5. The impact of co-morbidities on HAND

HIV, once an acute and catastrophic infection, has now become a chronic and manageable disease, with advances made in diagnosis and treatment. These changes are reflected in the increases in life expectancy from 5 years to up to the projected 50 years from the time of diagnosis. However, with the increased lifespan, co-morbidities, such as chronic co-infections, substance abuse, and aging have become major contributors to HAND persistence, and need to be addressed for successful evaluation and treatment of HAND.

The compromised immune system in an HIV-infected individual increases the risk of opportunistic infections in the CNS, much like that observed in the peripheral tissue. Most commonly observed infections, CNS toxoplasmosis, cryptococcosis, CNS tuberculosis, and cytomegalovirus encephalitis can be treated successfully by a combination of antimicrobials, antiviral and antiretroviral drugs. However, there are several other viral agents that can either directly target or indirectly compromise CNS, and cannot be readily managed by antiretroviral drugs or chemotherapeutics. One important virus with serious complications in HAND patients is JC virus, the causative agent of progressive multifocal leukoencephelopathy (PML). While approximately 60-80% of adults globally are seropositive for JC virus, it leads to the development of PML mostly in individuals who are immuno-compromised, either due to an underlying cancer or immunosuppressive treatment, or who are HIV-positive. The current incidence of PML in HIV patients is 3%. Studies have shown that JC virus can traffic across the BBB within the B cells, can enter the CNS as a free virus, or can infect brain vascular endothelial cells. Once in the CNS, JC virus causes the lytic infection of oligodendrocytes, and results in multifocal demyelination in multiple regions of the white matter. Thus, PML may exacerbate white matter loss that may already be occurring in HAND patients. Further, the most efficient, however limited, treatment for PML, which is immune restoration with aggressive antiretroviral therapy, can potentiate immune reconstitution inflammatory syndrome (IRIS). IRIS, a T-cell mediated encephalitis, can precipitate further injury and worsening of neurological symptoms. While fatality due to PML in HIV-infected individuals can be as high as 50%, the number of cases with non-lethal PML is increasing and PML may be contributing to the persistence of HIV-associated neurological complications.

Hepatitis B and C (HBV and HCV) are also commonly found in HIV-infected individuals due to the shared risk factors of contracting the virus. While these viruses are not thought to target the primary cells of the CNS, a recent study has reported the presence of HCV antigens in astrocytes and the cells of the macrophage/microglial lineage in the human brain. Additionally, there is limited evidence suggesting that HCV core protein might be detrimental to neurons *in vitro* and *in vivo*. Further, several studies have suggested that HCV and HIV can potentiate each other's replication. Currently, there is no conclusive data regarding a possible correlation between HCV presence in the CNS and the neurocognitive deficits in HAND patients. However, the potential implications of HCV infection in the CNS are at least three-fold. First, HCV co-infection can hinder the efforts to suppress HIV replication in the CNS. Second, weakened immune system function secondary to HCV will negatively impact subsequent alleviation of neurocognitive functions. Finally, compromised functioning of CNS support cells, mainly astrocytes, secondary to concomitant HCV infection will augment the neuroinflammatory environment with a negative impact on neuronal health. These implications may underlie the evidence that suggests that viral suppression and CD4+ cell recovery is not as successful in the presence of HCV, and might partially explain the sporadic data suggesting that worse neurocognitive impairment is observed in HIV-HCV co-infected patients [184].

Illicit drug use, as well as alcohol abuse, put HIV-positive patients at a greater risk for HAND [6, 218-224]. The prevalence of HIV infection is 11-17% among illicit drug users, and methamphetamine (METH) is among the most frequently abused drug with well-known toxic effects on the BBB and in the CNS [220]. HIV-infected patients using METH exhibit more neurocognitive deficits, compared to those not using METH. These findings are likely due to the effects of METH on several fronts in the CNS. First, extensive studies have conclusively shown that METH alters the BBB permeability through direct damage to the BMECs, which in turn can augment HIV access to the CNS. Additionally, METH can exert neurotoxic effects in the CNS through oxidative stress and mitochondrial dysfunction [184], and precipitate further synaptic and neuronal damage. METH may also interfere with the expected benefits of ART in several ways. Most importantly, studies have shown that altered patient behavior due to METH use can interfere with drug adherence. Secondly, altered BBB function in a patient using METH can potentially alter antiretroviral access to the CNS, hindering efforts to establish an efficient regimen with limited side effects.

6. Aging and HAND

The widespread use of ART has drastically decreased the incidence of AIDS-related complications and improved the long-term prognosis of HIV-positive individuals. Currently, 30% of the HIV-positive population in the United States is over the age of 50,and by 2015 it is estimated that more than 50% will be over the age of 50 [225, 226]. Despite this remarkable development, the life expectancy for ART-treated HIV-positive individuals remains 10-30 years less than that of uninfected individuals [227]. Given the rapid global expansion of this population, it has become increasingly important to understand the risk factors that lie at the intersection of HIV, ART, and aging.

Older HIV-positive patients, including those treated with ART, are at increased risk for systemic diseases including atherosclerosis, liver and kidney failure, cancer, and osteoporosis [227, 228]. The aging brain may also be more vulnerable to the effects of HIV as older adults display an increased susceptibility to HAND, and emerging evidence suggests an increased prevalence of neurodegenerative diseases, including Alzheimer and Parkinson, in this patient population [229, 230]. It remains unclear if the increased prevalence of HAND is a result of HIV and related comorbidities, including hypertension, insulin resistance, and lipodystrophy, or other confounding factors such as immunosenescence and ART toxicities, all of which are likely to impact CNS disease progression in older HIV-positive individuals [231, 232].

Antiretroviral therapy effectively limits HIV disease progression, maintains patients in a state of partial immune competence, and arrests subjects in a pre-symptomatic state [233]. However, despite the ability of ART to reduce plasma HIV RNA to undetectable levels, HIV-positive individuals remain at higher risk for opportunistic illnesses and premature death [234, 235]. Thus, ART may reduce, but does not appear to eliminate, premature and/or accelerated aging in HIV-infected individuals. This may be attributed to many factors including drug toxicity and slower immune recovery following ART initiation in older patients, compared to younger adults [236]. Furthermore, advanced age has been linked to decreased production of T cells, B cells, and cytokines as well as to chronic immune activation, the latter of which may be linked to the breakdown of gut-associated lymphoid tissue (GALT) and to the elevated levels of systemic lipopolysaccharide (LPS) [237, 238].

Older patients also display a dampened recovery of CD4 cells following treatment with ART, which may increase their risk for systemic diseases ranging from heart disease to cancer [238]. Thus, it is not surprising that advanced age at seroconversion and/or onset of ART treatment is considered a major risk factor for severe HIV disease [239, 240]. Goetz, et al. performed a retrospective study on HIV-positive patients receiving ART treatment at the Veteran's Administration Greater Los Angeles Medical center between 1996 and 1999, and found that for every 10 years of additional age at the onset of ART treatment, the rate of CD4 cell replenishment decreased by 35 cells per microliter of blood [241]. Yet, despite the obvious benefits of beginning ART treatment in asymptomatic HIV-positive individuals, there remain significant concerns for initiating drug therapy sooner than necessary and how this may negatively impact drug toxicity, long-term patient outcome, and the evolution of drug resistant strains of HIV [240, 242]. Based on the updated recommendations for treatment initiation, as mentioned previously, all HIV-infected individuals will be put on ART regimen upon diagnosis, and the impact of this approach on older patients will be revealing.

Lower CD4 count, in addition to advanced age, also places older patients at a nearly fourfold higher risk for liver-related mortality compared to younger patients [243]. This risk is exacerbated by other factors commonly afflicting ART-treated, HIV-positive individuals including diabetes, alcohol abuse, as well as antiretroviral and cholesterol drug toxicity [243]. Among all non-AIDS-related complications, liver disease is the primary cause of death in

HIV-positive patients [243]. In addition, older HIV-positive individuals are at increased risk for frailty, bone loss and non-AIDS related cancers [244, 245]. It remains unclear if HIV itself places older individuals at higher risk for heart disease compared to older, HIV-negative individuals, though specific classes of antiretrovirals, especially protease inhibitors, have been linked to atherosclerosis [237, 246, 247].

The CNS is particularly susceptible to the synergistic neurodegenerative effects of HIV and aging. Several studies have demonstrated that, compared to younger (age 20 to 39 years) cohorts, older HIV-positive individuals (age > 50 years) display decreased neurocognitive functioning in several areas including memory, psychomotor speed, and executive functions [225, 248, 249]. The persistence of HAND in individuals with an undetectable viral load and CD4 cell counts greater than 200/µL is not well understood and may be a result of aging-associated processes rendering the cells of the CNS more vulnerable.

Several recent neuroimaging studies have begun to address the structural, physiological, and functional changes in the CNS in the context of HIV and aging. Six MRI investigations that assessed the structural changes in the brains of older HIV-positive individuals between 1998 and 2012 found evidence of premature or accelerated aging characterized by significant brain atrophy in the basal ganglia, cerebellum, and frontal and temporal brain regions, when compared to seronegative controls [231]. However, several diffusion tensor imaging (DTI) studies found only normal, age-dependent changes in mean diffusion and fractional anisotropy, which reflects the directionality of water diffusion in the brain, and is greater along organized white matter tracts but decreased in pathologically damaged, disorganized tracts [231, 250-252].

Other studies have employed proton magnetic resonance spectroscopy (MRS) to assess the changes in brain metabolite levels that are indicative of neuronal damage and death or glial activation. Ernst and Chang demonstrated a five-fold acceleration of aging effects in a relatively young (mean age 36 years) ART-naïve, HIV-positive cohort, as compared to HIV-negative controls, as reflected by increased levels of glial activation markers, myoinositol (MI) and choline compounds (CHO), and a decrease in the neuronal marker, N-acetylaspartate (NAA) [253]. A recent multicenter MRS study of slightly older (ages 30-70], ART-treated HIV-positive individuals demonstrated elevated MI and CHO in all brain regions of patients with asymptomatic or mild neurocognitive impairment, but decreased levels of MI in those with dementia, which the authors interpreted as premature microglial senescence [231, 254]. In addition, this study found an age-dependent decrease in NAA in frontal white matter, but only in patients with HAD [254]. Thus, while ART-naïve HIV-positive patients show evidence of increased, age-dependent glial activation and neuronal damage leading to accelerated aging, ART-treated individuals show only signs of premature aging [231].

As mentioned previously, the clinical and pathological hallmarks of post-ART HAND differ from those in the pre-ART era. While HAD presented as a subcortical dementia afflicting the basal ganglia and white matter, some post-ART studies suggest the focus of neuroinflammation has shifted primarily to the hippocampus, even in effectively treated patients [255-257]. Furthermore, there is emerging evidence that pathologic similarities exist between HAND and some common neurodegenerative disorders such as Alzheimer Disease, which is characterized by the presence of extracellular beta amyloid (Aβ) plaque deposits, and intracellular neurofibrillary tangles composed of hyperphosphorylated Tau [228, 233, 258, 259]. *In vitro* work involving the viral protein Tat has demonstrated the ability of this viral protein to inhibit the activity of the Aβ-degrading enzyme, Neprilysin, and the ability to bind to the receptor for advanced glycation end products, all of which may promote Aβ accumulation in the CNS. Indeed, some individuals with HAND display CSF levels of Aβ42 comparable to those observed in AD patients [228, 260, 261]. However, a recent report utilizing the amyloid-binding, carbon 11-labeled Pittsburgh compound B (11C-PiB) and PET imaging found that irrespective of neurocognitive impairment, HIV-positive individuals showed no increase in 11C-PiB levels, highlighting a potential key difference between Aβ metabolism in HAND vs. AD despite some overlapping pathological features [258].

Among the studies underlining the similarities between HAND and AD, Esiri *et al.* were the first to report a predisposition to plaque formation in the brains of pre-ART HIV-positive individuals [262]. Such pathological changes have been observed in HIV-positive patients despite successful virologic control with ART, suggesting that antiretrovirals either cannot achieve therapeutic concentrations within the brain parenchyma, allowing for ongoing viral replication and neuroinflammation, or may have toxic effects that could facilitate neurodegeneration [263, 264]. To address the latter concern, several reports investigated differences in either phospho-tau or beta amyloid levels in ART-naïve vs. ART-treated individuals. Two groups independently reported elevated Aβ deposition in the hippocampus of ART-treated individuals compared to pre-ART patients, yet Anthony *et al.* reported only increased hyperphosphorylated tau, but no Aβ deposition in the hippocampus and entorhinal cortex of HIV-positive individuals [257, 259, 265]. To date, no group has reported concomitant phospho-tau and Aβ plaque depositions in the same brain samples from HIV-positive cohorts. Differences in patient age and ART-regimens, as well as the antibodies used to detect Aβ may account for the varied outcomes of these reports.

Importantly, the aforementioned studies highlight the potentially under-appreciated concern of antiretroviral-associated toxicity and its effect on neuropsychological outcomes in long-term ART-treated patients. As described earlier, ART drugs have been linked to wide-ranging, peripheral metabolic and neural disturbances that could themselves influence the progression of HAND and foretell potential mechanisms of toxicity in the CNS [246, 266-276]. While CNS effects of ART are poorly understood, Schweinsburg et al. demonstrated an association between NRTIs and decreased levels of frontal white matter NAA, which they attributed to NRTI-mediated mitochondrial dysfunction and depletion of cellular respiration [268]. Confounding the issue of direct CNS toxicity of antiretroviral medications is the variability in BBB permeability amongst different drug classes as determined by various physicochemical properties such as plasma protein binding, lipophilicity, and molecular size.

Although it is a widely held that ART regimens with higher CNS penetrance generally confer greater neuropsychological outcomes in HIV-positive individuals, numerous clinical studies have suggested these regimens may negatively impact cognition. In a prospective study, Marra et al. found a significant association between highly CNS-penetrant ART regimens and worse neurocognitive and motor performance, despite decreased CSF HIV RNA in a small HIV-positive cohort [181]. In addition, Robertson et al. reported an improvement in neuropsychological outcome in a cohort of patients with interrupted drug treatment [277]. Studies using SCID mice, which display neuropathological hallmarks similar to those associated with HIV, showed reduced viral load and astrogliosis following administration of ART, but no improvement in cognitive dysfunction [278]. Altogether, these studies reinforce an emerging hypothesis that antiretroviral drugs may be contributing to the rising prevalence of HAND in the aging HIV-positive population.

However, many clinical studies have demonstrated beneficial effects on neurocognitive functioning by ART regimens with high CPE scores [279, 280]. A cross-sectional study of 2636 adults from the AIDS Clinical Trials Group Longitudinal Linked Randomized Trials (ALLRT cohort), on effective ART for at least 6 weeks showed better neurocognitive performance in individuals receiving ART medications with higher CPE scores [281]. In some cases, participants required more than 3 antiretrovirals to treat HIV in the CNS. Letendre et al. demonstrated improvements in cognition over a 15-week period in patients beginning ART with higher CPE ART regimens [282]. Another recent investigation utilized MRS imaging to investigate the effect of different CPE ART regimens with different CPE scores on changes in brain NAA metabolite levels. Over 48 weeks, HIV-positive, ART-naïve individuals receiving the regimens with highest CPE scores displayed the highest increases in NAA levels, and showed the greatest improvement in a battery of neuropsychological tests [283]. These studies suggest that ART medications with higher CNS penetrance may have a neuroprotective effect in successfully treated HIV-positive adults. However, given the well-characterized toxicities of ART medications in the periphery, and the potential impact of related co-morbidities on CNS pathology, it may be necessary to consider adjunctive therapies to minimize the synergistic effects of ART and aging in HIV-positive individuals.

7. Summary

The advent of ART has profoundly changed the landscape of disease; however, neurocognitive impairments continue to be debilitating to patients with the expected life expectancy closer to that of the uninfected population. A better understanding and appreciation of the confounding factors has become more acute as the recent focus in the race to cure AIDS has shifted towards the eradication of latent viral reservoirs, including those in the CNS. It is imperative to anticipate and control the immune responses due to viral reactivation, the potential neurotoxicities of viral proteins in the brain parenchyma when latent viral progeny is activated, and the oxidative damage that may be precipitated by viral particles and the activated immune cells. These factors will be even more crucial to control in the aging brain with limited cognitive reserves.

Author details

Jennifer M. King, Brigid K. Jensen, Patrick J. Gannon and Cagla Akay*

*Address all correspondence to: akayc@upenn.edu

Department of Pathology, School of Dental Medicine, University of Pennsylvania, Philadelphia, USA

References

[1] Lindl KA, Marks DR, Kolson DL, Jordan-Sciutto KL. HIV-associated neurocognitive disorder: pathogenesis and therapeutic opportunities. J Neuroimmune Pharmacol. (Review). 2010 Sep;5 (3):294-309.

[2] Antinori A, Arendt G, Becker JT, Brew BJ, Byrd DA, Cherner M, et al. Updated research nosology for HIV-associated neurocognitive disorders. Neurology. 2007 Oct 30;69 (18):1789-99.

[3] Heaton RK, Clifford DB, Franklin DR, Jr., Woods SP, Ake C, Vaida F, et al. HIV-associated neurocognitive disorders persist in the era of potent antiretroviral therapy: CHARTER Study. Neurology. 2010 Dec 7;75 (23):2087-96.

[4] Dore GJ, Correll PK, Li Y, Kaldor JM, Cooper DA, Brew BJ. Changes to AIDS dementia complex in the era of highly active antiretroviral therapy. AIDS (London, England). 1999 Jul 9;13 (10):1249-53.

[5] Dore GJ, Li Y, McDonald A, Ree H, Kaldor JM. Impact of highly active antiretroviral therapy on individual AIDS-defining illness incidence and survival in Australia. Journal of acquired immune deficiency syndromes (1999). 2002 Apr 1;29 (4):388-95.

[6] Power C, Boisse L, Rourke S, Gill MJ. NeuroAIDS: an evolving epidemic. Can J Neurol Sci. 2009 May;36 (3):285-95.

[7] Price RW, Brew B, Sidtis J, Rosenblum M, Scheck AC, Cleary P. The brain in AIDS: central nervous system HIV-1 infection and AIDS dementia complex. Science. 1988;239:586-92.

[8] Gongvatana A, Schweinsburg BC, Taylor MJ, Theilmann RJ, Letendre SL, Alhassoon OM, et al. White matter tract injury and cognitive impairment in human immunodeficiency virus-infected individuals. J Neurovirol. 2009 Apr;15 (2):187-95.

[9] Thompson PM, Dutton RA, Hayashi KM, Toga AW, Lopez OL, Aizenstein HJ, et al. Thinning of the cerebral cortex visualized in HIV/AIDS reflects CD4+ T lymphocyte decline. Proc Natl Acad Sci U S A. 2005 Oct 25;102 (43):15647-52.

[10] Cohen RA, Harezlak J, Schifitto G, Hana G, Clark U, Gongvatana A, et al. Effects of nadir CD4 count and duration of human immunodeficiency virus infection on brain

volumes in the highly active antiretroviral therapy era. J Neurovirol. 2010 Feb;16 (1): 25-32.

[11] Ellis R. HIV and antiretroviral therapy: impact on the central nervous system. Prog Neurobiol. 2010 Jun;91 (2):185-7.

[12] Everall I, Vaida F, Khanlou N, Lazzaretto D, Achim C, Letendre S, et al. Cliniconeuropathologic correlates of human immunodeficiency virus in the era of antiretroviral therapy. J Neurovirol. 2009 Sep;15 (5-6):360-70.

[13] Everall IP, Heaton RK, Marcotte TD, Ellis RJ, McCutchan JA, Atkinson JH, et al. Cortical synaptic density is reduced in mild to moderate human immunodeficiency virus neurocognitive disorder. HNRC Group. HIV Neurobehavioral Research Center. Brain Pathol. 1999 Apr;9 (2):209-17.

[14] Masliah E, Heaton RK, Marcotte TD, Ellis RJ, Wiley CA, Mallory M, et al. Dendritic injury is a pathological substrate for human immunodeficiency virus-related cognitive disorders. HNRC Group. The HIV Neurobehavioral Research Center. Ann Neurol. 1997 Dec;42 (6):963-72.

[15] Zheng J, Thylin MR, Cotter RL, Lopez AL, Ghorpade A, Persidsky Y, et al. HIV-1 infected and immune competent mononuclear phagocytes induce quantitative alterations in neuronal dendritic arbor: relevance for HIV-1-associated dementia. Neurotox Res. 2001 Oct;3 (5):443-59.

[16] Gelman BB, Schuenke K. Brain aging in acquired immunodeficiency syndrome: increased ubiquitin-protein conjugate is correlated with decreased synaptic protein but not amyloid plaque accumulation. J Neurovirol. 2004 Apr;10 (2):98-108.

[17] Kolson DL, Sabnekar P, Baybis M, Crino PB. Gene expression in TUNEL-positive neurons in human immunodeficiency virus-infected brain. J Neurovirol. 2004;10 Suppl 1:102-7.

[18] Wiley CA, Achim CL, Hammond R, Love S, Masliah E, Radhakrishnan L, et al. Damage and repair of DNA in HIV encephalitis. J Neuropathol Exp Neurol. 2000 Nov;59 (11):955-65.

[19] Gonzalez-Scarano F, Martin-Garcia J. The neuropathogenesis of AIDS. Nat Rev Immunol. 2005 Jan;5 (1):69-81.

[20] Fauci AS. The human immunodeficiency virus: infectivity and mechanisms of pathogenesis. Science. 1988 Feb 5;239 (4840):617-22.

[21] Williams DW, Eugenin EA, Calderon TM, Berman JW. Monocyte maturation, HIV susceptibility, and transmigration across the blood brain barrier are critical in HIV neuropathogenesis. J Leukoc Biol. 2012 Mar;91 (3):401-15.

[22] Roberts TK, Buckner CM, Berman JW. Leukocyte transmigration across the blood-brain barrier: perspectives on neuroAIDS. Front Biosci. 2010;15:478-536.

[23] Liu NQ, Lossinsky AS, Popik W, Li X, Gujuluva C, Kriederman B, et al. Human immunodeficiency virus type 1 enters brain microvascular endothelia by macropinocytosis dependent on lipid rafts and the mitogen-activated protein kinase signaling pathway. J Virol. 2002 Jul;76 (13):6689-700.

[24] Gendelman HE, Lipton SA, Tardieu M, Bukrinsky MI, Nottet HS. The neuropathogenesis of HIV-1 infection. (see comment). (Review) (107 refs). 1994 Sep.

[25] Gonzalez-Scarano F, Martin-Garcia J. The neuropathogenesis of AIDS. (Review) (173 refs). 2005 Jan.

[26] Kaul M, Zheng J, Okamoto S, Gendelman HE, Lipton SA. HIV-1 infection and AIDS: consequences for the central nervous system. (Review) (199 refs). 2005 Aug.

[27] Carter CC, Onafuwa-Nuga A, McNamara LA, Riddell Jt, Bixby D, Savona MR, et al. HIV-1 infects multipotent progenitor cells causing cell death and establishing latent cellular reservoirs. Nat Med. 2010 Apr;16 (4):446-51.

[28] Hakre S, Chavez L, Shirakawa K, Verdin E. HIV latency: experimental systems and molecular models. FEMS Microbiol Rev. 2012 May;36 (3):706-16.

[29] Lafeuillade A. Eliminating the HIV reservoir. Curr HIV/AIDS Rep. 2012 Jun;9 (2): 121-31.

[30] Saleh S, Wightman F, Ramanayake S, Alexander M, Kumar N, Khoury G, et al. Expression and reactivation of HIV in a chemokine induced model of HIV latency in primary resting CD4+ T cells. Retrovirology. 2011;8:80.

[31] Vandergeeten C, Fromentin R, Chomont N. The role of cytokines in the establishment, persistence and eradication of the HIV reservoir. Cytokine Growth Factor Rev. 2012 Aug;23 (4-5):143-9.

[32] Wilen CB, Tilton JC, Doms RW. Molecular mechanisms of HIV entry. Adv Exp Med Biol. 2012;726:223-42.

[33] Devadas K, Hardegen NJ, Wahl LM, Hewlett IK, Clouse KA, Yamada KM, et al. Mechanisms for macrophage-mediated HIV-1 induction. J Immunol. 2004 Dec 1;173 (11):6735-44.

[34] Gorry PR, Ong C, Thorpe J, Bannwarth S, Thompson KA, Gatignol A, et al. Astrocyte infection by HIV-1: mechanisms of restricted virus replication, and role in the pathogenesis of HIV-1-associated dementia. Curr HIV Res. 2003 Oct;1 (4):463-73.

[35] Wraith DC, Nicholson LB. The adaptive immune system in diseases of the central nervous system. J Clin Invest. 2012 Apr 2;122 (4):1172-9.

[36] Ransohoff RM, Brown MA. Innate immunity in the central nervous system. J Clin Invest. 2012 Apr 2;122 (4):1164-71.

[37] Fairweather D, Cihakova D. Alternatively activated macrophages in infection and autoimmunity. J Autoimmun. 2009 Nov-Dec;33 (3-4):222-30.

[38] Fujiwara N, Kobayashi K. Macrophages in inflammation. Curr Drug Targets Inflamm Allergy. 2005 Jun;4 (3):281-6.

[39] Tesseur I, Wyss-Coray T. A role for TGF-beta signaling in neurodegeneration: evidence from genetically engineered models. Curr Alzheimer Res. 2006 Dec;3 (5): 505-13.

[40] Wahl SM, Allen JB, McCartney-Francis N, Morganti-Kossmann MC, Kossmann T, Ellingsworth L, et al. Macrophage- and astrocyte-derived transforming growth factor beta as a mediator of central nervous system dysfunction in acquired immune deficiency syndrome. J Exp Med. 1991 Apr 1;173 (4):981-91.

[41] Wahl SM. The role of transforming growth factor-beta in inflammatory processes. Immunol Res. 1991;10 (3-4):249-54.

[42] Johnson MD, Gold LI. Distribution of transforming growth factor-beta isoforms in human immunodeficiency virus-1 encephalitis. Hum Pathol. 1996 Jul;27 (7):643-9.

[43] Dhar A, Gardner J, Borgmann K, Wu L, Ghorpade A. Novel role of TGF-beta in differential astrocyte-TIMP-1 regulation: implications for HIV-1-dementia and neuroinflammation. J Neurosci Res. 2006 May 15;83 (7):1271-80.

[44] Samah B, Porcheray F, Dereuddre-Bosquet N, Gras G. Nerve growth factor stimulation promotes CXCL-12 attraction of monocytes but decreases human immunodeficiency virus replication in attracted population. J Neurovirol. 2009 Jan;15 (1):71-80.

[45] Meeker RB, Poulton W, Markovic-Plese S, Hall C, Robertson K. Protein changes in CSF of HIV-infected patients: evidence for loss of neuroprotection. J Neurovirol. (Research Support, N.I.H., Extramural). 2011 Jun;17 (3):258-73.

[46] Heath SL, Sabbaj S, Bansal A, Kilby JM, Goepfert PA. CD8 T-cell proliferative capacity is compromised in primary HIV-1 infection. Journal of acquired immune deficiency syndromes (1999). 2011 Mar;56 (3):213-21.

[47] Yadav A, Collman RG. CNS inflammation and macrophage/microglial biology associated with HIV-1 infection. J Neuroimmune Pharmacol. 2009 Dec;4 (4):430-47.

[48] Tozzi V, Balestra P, Bellagamba R, Corpolongo A, Salvatori MF, Visco-Comandini U, et al. Persistence of neuropsychologic deficits despite long-term highly active antiretroviral therapy in patients with HIV-related neurocognitive impairment: prevalence and risk factors. Journal of acquired immune deficiency syndromes (1999). 2007 Jun 1;45 (2):174-82.

[49] Yilmaz A, Price RW, Spudich S, Fuchs D, Hagberg L, Gisslen M. Persistent intrathecal immune activation in HIV-1-infected individuals on antiretroviral therapy. Journal of acquired immune deficiency syndromes (1999). 2008 Feb 1;47 (2):168-73.

[50] Yilmaz A, Fuchs D, Hagberg L, Nillroth U, Stahle L, Svensson J-O, et al. Cerebrospinal fluid HIV-1 RNA, intrathecal immunoactivation, and drug concentrations after

treatment with a combination of saquinavir, nelfinavir, and two nucleoside analogues: the M61022 study. BMC Infectious Diseases. 2006;6 (1):63.

[51] Edén A, Fuchs D, Hagberg L, Nilsson S, Spudich S, Svennerholm B, et al. HIV-1 Viral Escape in Cerebrospinal Fluid of Subjects on Suppressive Antiretroviral Treatment. Journal of Infectious Diseases. 2010 December 15, 2010;202 (12):1819-25.

[52] Hagberg L, Cinque P, Gisslen M, Brew B, Spudich S, Bestetti A, et al. Cerebrospinal fluid neopterin: an informative biomarker of central nervous system immune activation in HIV-1 infection. AIDS Research and Therapy. 2010;7 (1):15.

[53] Achim CL, Masliah E, Heyes MP, Sarnacki P, Hilty C, Baldwin M, et al. Macrophage Activation Factors
in the Brains of AIDS Patients. Journal of neuro-AIDS. 1996;1 (2):1-16.

[54] Achim CL, Wiley CA. Inflammation in AIDS and the role of the macrophage in brain pathology. Curr Opin Neurobiol. 1996;9 (3):221-5.

[55] Conant K, Garzino-Demo A, Nath A, McArthur JC, Halliday W, Power C, et al. Induction of monocyte chemoattractant protein-1 in HIV-1 Tat-stimulated astrocytes and elevation in AIDS dementia. Proc Natl Acad Sci U S A. 1998 Mar 17;95 (6): 3117-21.

[56] Gisolf EH, van Praag RM, Jurriaans S, Portegies P, Goudsmit J, Danner SA, et al. Increasing cerebrospinal fluid chemokine concentrations despite undetectable cerebrospinal fluid HIV RNA in HIV-1-infected patients receiving antiretroviral therapy. Journal of acquired immune deficiency syndromes (1999). 2000 Dec 15;25 (5):426-33.

[57] Sippy BD, Hofman FM, Wallach D, Hinton DR. Increased expression of tumor necrosis factor-alpha receptors in the brains of patients with AIDS. J Acquir Immune Defic Syndr Hum Retrovirol. 1995 Dec 15;10 (5):511-21.

[58] Tomkowicz B, Lee C, Ravyn V, Cheung R, Ptasznik A, Collman RG. The Src kinase Lyn is required for CCR5 signaling in response to MIP-1beta and R5 HIV-1 gp120 in human macrophages. Blood. 2006 Aug 15;108 (4):1145-50.

[59] Lee C, Tomkowicz B, Freedman BD, Collman RG. HIV-1 gp120-induced TNF-(alpha) production by primary human macrophages is mediated by phosphatidylinositol-3 (PI-3) kinase and mitogen-activated protein (MAP) kinase pathways. J Leukoc Biol. 2005 Oct;78 (4):1016-23.

[60] Chihara T, Hashimoto M, Osman A, Hiyoshi-Yoshidomi Y, Suzu I, Chutiwitoonchai N, et al. HIV-1 proteins preferentially activate anti-inflammatory M2-type macrophages. J Immunol. 2012 Apr 15;188 (8):3620-7.

[61] Turchan-Cholewo J, Dimayuga VM, Gupta S, Gorospe RM, Keller JN, Bruce-Keller AJ. NADPH oxidase drives cytokine and neurotoxin release from microglia and macrophages in response to HIV-Tat. Antioxid Redox Signal. 2009 Feb;11 (2):193-204.

[62] Pu H, Tian J, Flora G, Lee YW, Nath A, Hennig B, et al. HIV-1 Tat protein upregulates inflammatory mediators and induces monocyte invasion into the brain. Mol Cell Neurosci. 2003 Sep;24 (1):224-37.

[63] Agrawal L, Louboutin JP, Marusich E, Reyes BA, Van Bockstaele EJ, Strayer DS. Dopaminergic neurotoxicity of HIV-1 gp120: reactive oxygen species as signaling intermediates. Brain Res. 2010 Jan 8;1306:116-30.

[64] Louboutin JP, Agrawal L, Reyes BA, Van Bockstaele EJ, Strayer DS. Protecting neurons from HIV-1 gp120-induced oxidant stress using both localized intracerebral and generalized intraventricular administration of antioxidant enzymes delivered by SV40-derived vectors. Gene Ther. 2007 Dec;14 (23):1650-61.

[65] Agrawal L, Louboutin JP, Reyes BA, Van Bockstaele EJ, Strayer DS. HIV-1 Tat neurotoxicity: a model of acute and chronic exposure, and neuroprotection by gene delivery of antioxidant enzymes. Neurobiol Dis. 2012 Feb;45 (2):657-70.

[66] Gannon P, Khan MZ, Kolson DL. Current understanding of HIV-associated neurocognitive disorders pathogenesis. Curr Opin Neurol. (Research Support, N.I.H., ExtramuralReview). 2011 Jun;24 (3):275-83.

[67] Rao JS, Kim HW, Kellom M, Greenstein D, Chen M, Kraft AD, et al. Increased neuroinflammatory and arachidonic acid cascade markers, and reduced synaptic proteins, in brain of HIV-1 transgenic rats. J Neuroinflammation. 2011;8:101.

[68] Kusao I, Shiramizu B, Liang CY, Grove J, Agsalda M, Troelstrup D, et al. Cognitive performance related to HIV-1-infected monocytes. J Neuropsychiatry Clin Neurosci. 2012 Dec 1;24 (1):71-80.

[69] Rostasy K, Monti L, Yiannoutsos C, Wu J, Bell J, Hedreen J, et al. NFkappaB activation, TNF-alpha expression, and apoptosis in the AIDS-Dementia-Complex. J Neurovirol. 2000 Dec;6 (6):537-43.

[70] Pemberton LA, Stone E, Price P, van Bockxmeer F, Brew BJ. The relationship between ApoE, TNFA, IL1a, IL1b and IL12b genes and HIV-1-associated dementia. HIV Med. 2008 Oct;9 (8):677-80.

[71] Lichtfuss GF, Cheng WJ, Farsakoglu Y, Paukovics G, Rajasuriar R, Velayudham P, et al. Virologically Suppressed HIV Patients Show Activation of NK Cells and Persistent Innate Immune Activation. J Immunol. 2012 Aug 1;189 (3):1491-9.

[72] Goldberg SH, van der Meer P, Hesselgesser J, Jaffer S, Kolson DL, Albright AV, et al. CXCR3 expression in human central nervous system diseases. Neuropathol Appl Neurobiol. 2001 Apr;27 (2):127-38.

[73] Letendre S, Zheng J, Kaul M, Yiannoutsos C, Ellis R, Taylor M, et al. Chemokines in cerebrospinal fluid correlate with cerebral metabolite patterns in HIV-infected individuals. Journal of NeuroVirology. 2011;17 (1):63-9.

[74] Martin-Garcia J, Kolson DL, Gonzalez-Scarano F. Chemokine receptors in the brain: their role in HIV infection and pathogenesis. AIDS (London, England). 2002 Sep 6;16 (13):1709-30.

[75] van der Meer P, Ulrich AM, Gonzalez-Scarano F, Lavi E. Immunohistochemical analysis of CCR2, CCR3, CCR5, and CXCR4 in the human brain: potential mechanisms for HIV dementia. Exp Mol Pathol. 2000 Dec;69 (3):192-201.

[76] Dhillon NK, Williams R, Callen S, Zien C, Narayan O, Buch S. Roles of MCP-1 in development of HIV-dementia. Front Biosci. 2008;13:3913-8.

[77] Monteiro de Almeida S, Letendre S, Zimmerman J, Lazzaretto D, McCutchan A, Ellis R. Dynamics of monocyte chemoattractant protein type one (MCP-1) and HIV viral load in human cerebrospinal fluid and plasma. Journal of neuroimmunology. 2005 Dec;169 (1-2):144-52.

[78] Cartier L, Dubois-Dauphin M, Hartley O, Irminger-Finger I, Krause KH. Chemokine-induced cell death in CCR5-expressing neuroblastoma cells. Journal of neuroimmunology. 2003 Dec;145 (1-2):27-39.

[79] Kraft-Terry SD, Stothert AR, Buch S, Gendelman HE. HIV-1 neuroimmunity in the era of antiretroviral therapy. Neurobiol Dis. 2010 Mar;37 (3):542-8.

[80] Alirezaei M, Watry DD, Flynn CF, Kiosses WB, Masliah E, Williams BR, et al. Human immunodeficiency virus-1/surface glycoprotein 120 induces apoptosis through RNA-activated protein kinase signaling in neurons. J Neurosci. 2007 Oct 10;27 (41): 11047-55.

[81] O'Donnell LA, Agrawal A, Jordan-Sciutto KL, Dichter MA, Lynch DR, Kolson DL. Human immunodeficiency virus (HIV)-induced neurotoxicity: roles for the NMDA receptor subtypes. J Neurosci. 2006 Jan 18;26 (3):981-90.

[82] Abdulle S, Hagberg L, Gisslen M. Effects of antiretroviral treatment on blood-brain barrier integrity and intrathecal immunoglobulin production in neuroasymptomatic HIV-1-infected patients. HIV Med. 2005 May;6 (3):164-9.

[83] Kamat A, Lyons JL, Misra V, Uno H, Morgello S, Singer EJ, et al. Monocyte Activation Markers in Cerebrospinal Fluid Associated With Impaired Neurocognitive Testing in Advanced HIV Infection. Journal of acquired immune deficiency syndromes (1999). 2012 Jul 1;60 (3):234-43.

[84] Schellenberg AE, Buist R, Del Bigio MR, Khorooshi R, Toft-Hansen H, Owens T, et al. Blood-brain barrier disruption in CCL2 transgenic mice during pertussis toxin-induced brain inflammation. Fluids and barriers of the CNS. 2012 Apr 30;9 (1):10.

[85] Eugenin EA, Osiecki K, Lopez L, Goldstein H, Calderon TM, Berman JW. CCL2/monocyte chemoattractant protein-1 mediates enhanced transmigration of human immunodeficiency virus (HIV)-infected leukocytes across the blood-brain barrier: a potential mechanism of HIV-CNS invasion and NeuroAIDS. J Neurosci. (Compara-

tive StudyResearch Support, N.I.H., ExtramuralResearch Support, Non-U.S. Gov't). 2006 Jan 25;26 (4):1098-106.

[86] Roberts TK, Eugenin EA, Lopez L, Romero IA, Weksler BB, Couraud PO, et al. CCL2 disrupts the adherens junction: implications for neuroinflammation. Lab Invest. 2012 Aug;92 (8):1213-33.

[87] Lu SM, Tremblay ME, King IL, Qi J, Reynolds HM, Marker DF, et al. HIV-1 Tat-induced microgliosis and synaptic damage via interactions between peripheral and central myeloid cells. PLoS One. 2011;6 (9):e23915.

[88] Markowitz AJ, White MG, Kolson DL, Jordan-Sciutto KL. Cellular interplay between neurons and glia: toward a comprehensive mechanism for excitotoxic neuronal loss in neurodegeneration. Cellscience. 2007 Jul 27;4 (1):111-46.

[89] Benos DJ, Hahn BH, Bubien JK, Ghosh SK, Mashburn NA, Chaikin MA, et al. Envelope glycoprotein gp120 of human immunodeficiency virus type 1 alters ion transport in astrocytes: implications for AIDS dementia complex. Proc Natl Acad Sci U S A. 1994 Jan 18;91 (2):494-8.

[90] Kolson DL, Buchhalter J, Collman R, Hellmig B, Farrell CF, Debouck C, et al. HIV-1 Tat alters normal organization of neurons and astrocytes in primary rodent brain cell cultures: RGD sequence dependence. AIDS Res Hum Retroviruses. 1993 Jul;9 (7): 677-85.

[91] Reddy PV, Gandhi N, Samikkannu T, Saiyed Z, Agudelo M, Yndart A, et al. HIV-1 gp120 induces antioxidant response element-mediated expression in primary astrocytes: Role in HIV associated neurocognitive disorder. Neurochem Int. 2011 Jul 3.

[92] Shukla V, Mishra SK, Pant HC. Oxidative stress in neurodegeneration. Adv Pharmacol Sci. 2011;2011:572634.

[93] Reynolds A, Laurie C, Mosley RL, Gendelman HE. Oxidative stress and the pathogenesis of neurodegenerative disorders. Int Rev Neurobiol. 2007;82:297-325.

[94] Melo A, Monteiro L, Lima RM, Oliveira DM, Cerqueira MD, El-Bacha RS. Oxidative stress in neurodegenerative diseases: mechanisms and therapeutic perspectives. Oxid Med Cell Longev. 2011;2011:467180.

[95] Ramsey C, Glass CA, Montgomery MB, Lindl KA, Ritson GP, Chia LA, Hamilton RL, Chu CT, Jordan-Sciutto KL. Expression of Nrf2 in Neurodegenerative Diseases. J Neuropathol Exp Neurol. 2007;66 (1):75-85.

[96] Lipton S. Update on current models of HIV-related neuronal injury: platelet-activating factor, arachidonic acid, and nitric oxide. Adv Neuroimmunol. 1994;4 (3):181-8.

[97] Mondal D, Pradhan L, Ali M, Agrawal KC. HAART drugs induce oxidative stress in human endothelial cells and increase endothelial recruitment of mononuclear cells: exacerbation by inflammatory cytokines and amelioration by antioxidants. Cardiovasc Toxicol. 2004;4 (3):287-302.

[98]   Lagathu C, Eustace B, Prot M, Frantz D, Gu Y, Bastard JP, et al. Some HIV antiretro-
       virals increase oxidative stress and alter chemokine, cytokine or adiponectin produc-
       tion in human adipocytes and macrophages. Antivir Ther. 2007;12 (4):489-500.

[99]   Chandra S, Mondal D, Agrawal KC. HIV-1 protease inhibitor induced oxidative
       stress suppresses glucose stimulated insulin release: protection with thymoquinone.
       Exp Biol Med (Maywood). 2009 Apr;234 (4):442-53.

[100] Walsh KA, Megyesi JF, Wilson JX, Crukley J, Laubach VE, Hammond RR. Antioxi-
       dant protection from HIV-1 gp120-induced neuroglial toxicity. J Neuroinflammation.
       2004 May 27;1 (1):8.

[101] Cherry CL, Duncan AJ, Mackie KF, Wesselingh SL, Brew BJ. A Report on the Effect
       of Commencing Enfuvirtide on Peripheral Neuropathy. AIDS Research and Human
       Retroviruses. 2008;24 (8):1027-30.

[102] Blas-Garcia A, Apostolova N, Esplugues JV. Oxidative stress and mitochondrial im-
       pairment after treatment with anti-HIV drugs: clinical implications. Curr Pharm Des.
       2011 Dec 1;17 (36):4076-86.

[103] Hulgan T, Morrow J, D'Aquila RT, Raffanti S, Morgan M, Rebeiro P, et al. Oxidant
       stress is increased during treatment of human immunodeficiency virus infection.
       Clin Infect Dis. 2003 Dec 15;37 (12):1711-7.

[104] Mandas A, Iorio EL, Congiu MG, Balestrieri C, Mereu A, Cau D, et al. Oxidative im-
       balance in HIV-1 infected patients treated with antiretroviral therapy. Journal of bio-
       medicine & biotechnology. 2009;2009:749575.

[105] Calkins M, Johnson DA, Townsend JA, Vargas MR, Dowell JA, Williamson TP, Kraft
       AD, Lee JM, Li J, Johnson JA. The Nrf2/ARE Pathway as a Potential Therapeutic Tar-
       get in Neurodegenerative Disease. Antiox Redox Sig. 2009;11 (3):497-508.

[106] Sonnerborg A, Carlin G, Akerlund B, Jarstrand C. Increased production of malon-
       dialdehyde in patients with HIV infection. Scand J Infect Dis. 1988;20 (3):287-90.

[107] Moore K, Roberts LJ, 2nd. Measurement of lipid peroxidation. Free radical research.
       1998 Jun;28 (6):659-71.

[108] McLemore JL, Beeley P, Thorton K, Morrisroe K, Blackwell W, Dasgupta A. Rapid
       automated determination of lipid hydroperoxide concentrations and total antioxi-
       dant status of serum samples from patients infected with HIV: elevated lipid hydro-
       peroxide concentrations and depleted total antioxidant capacity of serum samples.
       Am J Clin Pathol. 1998 Mar;109 (3):268-73.

[109] Favier A, Sappey C, Leclerc P, Faure P, Micoud M. Antioxidant status and lipid per-
       oxidation in patients infected with HIV. Chem Biol Interact. 1994 Jun;91 (2-3):165-80.

[110] Allard JP, Aghdassi E, Chau J, Salit I, Walmsley S. Oxidative stress and plasma anti-
       oxidant micronutrients in humans with HIV infection. Am J Clin Nutr. 1998 Jan;67
       (1):143-7.

[111] Malvy DJ, Richard MJ, Arnaud J, Favier A, Amedee-Manesme O. Relationship of plasma malondialdehyde, vitamin E and antioxidant micronutrients to human immunodeficiency virus-1 seropositivity. Clin Chim Acta. 1994 Jan 14;224 (1):89-94.

[112] Walmsley SL, Winn LM, Harrison ML, Uetrecht JP, Wells PG. Oxidative stress and thiol depletion in plasma and peripheral blood lymphocytes from HIV-infected patients: toxicological and pathological implications. AIDS (London, England). 1997 Nov 15;11 (14):1689-97.

[113] Jareno EJ, Bosch-Morell F, Fernandez-Delgado R, Donat J, Romero FJ. Serum malondialdehyde in HIV seropositive children. Free Radic Biol Med. 1998 Feb;24 (3):503-6.

[114] Repetto M, Reides C, Gomez Carretero ML, Costa M, Griemberg G, Llesuy S. Oxidative stress in blood of HIV infected patients. Clin Chim Acta. 1996 Nov 29;255 (2): 107-17.

[115] Sacktor N, Haughey N, Cutler R, Tamara A, Turchan J, Pardo C, Vargas D, Nath A. Novel markers of oxidative stress in actively progressive HIV dementia. Journal of neuroimmunology. 2004;157:176-84.

[116] Haughey NJ, Cutler RG, Tamara A, McArthur JC, Vargas DL, Pardo CA, et al. Perturbation of sphingolipid metabolism and ceramide production in HIV-dementia. Ann Neurol. 2004 Feb;55 (2):257-67.

[117] Turchan J, Pocernich CB, Gairola C, Chauhan A, Schifitto G, Butterfield DA, Buch S, Narayan O, Sinai A, Geiger J, Berger JR, Elford H, Nath A. Oxidative stress in HIV demented patients and protection ex vivo with novel antioxidants. Neurology. 2003;60:307-14.

[118] Suresh DR, Annam V, Pratibha K, Prasad BV. Total antioxidant capacity--a novel early bio-chemical marker of oxidative stress in HIV infected individuals. J Biomed Sci. 2009;16:61.

[119] Haughey NJ, Steiner J, Nath A, McArthur JC, Sacktor N, Pardo C, et al. Converging roles for sphingolipids and cell stress in the progression of neuro-AIDS. Front Biosci. 2008;13:5120-30.

[120] Droge W, Eck HP, Mihm S. Oxidant-antioxidant status in human immunodeficiency virus infection. Methods Enzymol. 1994;233:594-601.

[121] Ogunro PS, Ogungbamigbe TO, Elemie PO, Egbewale BE, Adewole TA. Plasma selenium concentration and glutathione peroxidase activity in HIV-1/AIDS infected patients: a correlation with the disease progression. Niger Postgrad Med J. 2006 Mar;13 (1):1-5.

[122] Dworkin BM, Rosenthal WS, Wormser GP, Weiss L. Selenium deficiency in the acquired immunodeficiency syndrome. JPEN J Parenter Enteral Nutr. 1986 Jul-Aug;10 (4):405-7.

[123] Sudfeld CR, Wang M, Aboud S, Giovannucci EL, Mugusi FM, Fawzi WW. Vitamin D and HIV Progression among Tanzanian Adults Initiating Antiretroviral Therapy. PLoS ONE. 2012;7 (6):e40036.

[124] Srinivas A, Dias BF. Antioxidants in HIV positive children. Indian J Pediatr. 2008 Apr;75 (4):347-50.

[125] Bilbis LS, Idowu DB, Saidu Y, Lawal M, Njoku CH. Serum levels of antioxidant vitamins and mineral elements of human immunodeficiency virus positive subjects in Sokoto, Nigeria. Ann Afr Med. 2010 Oct-Dec;9 (4):235-9.

[126] Oliveira KF, Cunha DF, Weffort VR. Analysis of serum and supplemented vitamin C and oxidative stress in HIV-infected children and adolescents. J Pediatr (Rio J). 2011 Nov-Dec;87 (6):517-22.

[127] Delmas-Beauvieux MC, Peuchant E, Couchouron A, Constans J, Sergeant C, Simonoff M, et al. The enzymatic antioxidant system in blood and glutathione status in human immunodeficiency virus (HIV)-infected patients: effects of supplementation with selenium or beta-carotene. Am J Clin Nutr. 1996 Jul;64 (1):101-7.

[128] Boven LA, Gomes L, Hery C, Gray F, Verhoef J, Portegies P, et al. Increased peroxynitrite activity in AIDS dementia complex: implications for the neuropathogenesis of HIV-1 infection. J Immunol. (Research Support, Non-U.S. Gov't). 1999 Apr 1;162 (7): 4319-27.

[129] Aukrust P, Svardal AM, Muller F, Lunden B, Berge RK, Ueland PM, et al. Increased levels of oxidized glutathione in CD4+ lymphocytes associated with disturbed intracellular redox balance in human immunodeficiency virus type 1 infection. Blood. 1995 Jul 1;86 (1):258-67.

[130] Buhl R, Jaffe HA, Holroyd KJ, Wells FB, Mastrangeli A, Saltini C, et al. Systemic glutathione deficiency in symptom-free HIV-seropositive individuals. Lancet. 1989 Dec 2;2 (8675):1294-8.

[131] Jaruga P, Jaruga B, Olczak A, Halota W, Olinski R. Oxidative DNA base damage in lymphocytes of HIV-infected drug users. Free radical research. 1999 Sep;31 (3): 197-200.

[132] Roc AC, Ances BM, Chawla S, Korczykowski M, Wolf RL, Kolson DL, et al. Detection of Human Immunodeficiency Virus Induced Inflammation and Oxidative Stress in Lenticular Nuclei With Magnetic Resonance Spectroscopy Despite Antiretroviral Therapy. 2007. p. 1249-57.

[133] Wanchu A, Rana SV, Pallikkuth S, Sachdeva RK. Short communication: oxidative stress in HIV-infected individuals: a cross-sectional study. AIDS Res Hum Retroviruses. 2009 Dec;25 (12):1307-11.

[134] Flourie F, Arab K, Gagnieu MC, Tardy JC, Jeanblanc F, Livrozet JM, et al. (Redox status in HIV+ patients under HAART). Ann Biol Clin (Paris). 2004 Nov-Dec;62 (6): 713-5.

[135] Gil L, Tarinas A, Hernandez D, Riveron BV, Perez D, Tapanes R, et al. Altered oxidative stress indexes related to disease progression marker in human immunodeficiency virus infected patients with antiretroviral therapy. Biomed Pharmacother. 2010 Sep 25.

[136] Ibeh BO, Obidoa O, Nwuke C. Lipid Peroxidation Correlates with HIVmRNA in Serodiscordant Heterosexual HIVpartners of Nigerian Origin. Indian J Clin Biochem. 2011 Jul;26 (3):249-56.

[137] Ibeh BO, Emeka-Nwabunnia IK. Increased oxidative stress condition found in different stages of HIV disease in patients undergoing antiretroviral therapy in Umuahia (Nigeria). Immunopharmacol Immunotoxicol. 2012 Apr 28.

[138] Masia M, Padilla S, Bernal E, Almenar MV, Molina J, Hernandez I, et al. Influence of antiretroviral therapy on oxidative stress and cardiovascular risk: a prospective cross-sectional study in HIV-infected patients. Clin Ther. 2007 Jul;29 (7):1448-55.

[139] Ngondi JL, Oben J, Forkah DM, Etame LH, Mbanya D. The effect of different combination therapies on oxidative stress markers in HIV infected patients in Cameroon. AIDS Res Ther. 2006;3:19.

[140] Hurwitz BE, Klimas NG, Llabre MM, Maher KJ, Skyler JS, Bilsker MS, et al. HIV, metabolic syndrome X, inflammation, oxidative stress, and coronary heart disease risk : role of protease inhibitor exposure. Cardiovasc Toxicol. 2004;4 (3):303-16.

[141] Stephensen CB, Marquis GS, Jacob RA, Kruzich LA, Douglas SD, Wilson CM. Vitamins C and E in adolescents and young adults with HIV infection. Am J Clin Nutr. 2006 Apr;83 (4):870-9.

[142] Stephensen CB, Marquis GS, Douglas SD, Kruzich LA, Wilson CM. Glutathione, glutathione peroxidase, and selenium status in HIV-positive and HIV-negative adolescents and young adults. Am J Clin Nutr. 2007 Jan;85 (1):173-81.

[143] Sundaram M, Saghayam S, Priya B, Venkatesh KK, Balakrishnan P, Shankar EM, et al. Changes in antioxidant profile among HIV-infected individuals on generic highly active antiretroviral therapy in southern India. Int J Infect Dis. 2008 Nov;12 (6):e61-6.

[144] Padmanabhan V, Rai K, Hegde AM, Shetty S. Total antioxidant capacity of saliva in children with HIV. J Clin Pediatr Dent. 2010 Summer;34 (4):347-50.

[145] Awodele O, Olayemi SO, Nwite JA, Adeyemo TA. Investigation of the levels of oxidative stress parameters in HIV and HIV-TB co-infected patients. J Infect Dev Ctries. 2012 Jan;6 (1):79-85.

[146] Paul S, Bogdanov MB, Matson WR, Metakis L, Jacobs J, Beal MF. Urinary 8-hydroxy-2'-deoxyguanosine, a metabolite of oxidized DNA, is not elevated in HIV patients on combination antiretroviral therapy. Free radical research. 2003 May;37 (5): 499-502.

[147] Zhang Y, Wang M, Li H, Zhang H, Shi Y, Wei F, et al. Accumulation of nuclear and mitochondrial DNA damage in the frontal cortex cells of patients with HIV-associated neurocognitive disorders. Brain Res. 2012 Jun 6;1458:1-11.

[148] Edeas MA, Emerit I, Khalfoun Y, Lazizi Y, Cernjavski L, Levy A, et al. Clastogenic factors in plasma of HIV-1 infected patients activate HIV-1 replication in vitro: inhibition by superoxide dismutase. Free Radic Biol Med. 1997;23 (4):571-8.

[149] Kimura T, Kameoka M, Ikuta K. Amplification of superoxide anion generation in phagocytic cells by HIV-1 infection. FEBS letters. 1993 Jul 12;326 (1-3):232-6.

[150] Mollace V, Salvemini D, Riley DP, Muscoli C, Iannone M, Granato T, et al. The contribution of oxidative stress in apoptosis of human-cultured astroglial cells induced by supernatants of HIV-1-infected macrophages. J Leukoc Biol. 2002 Jan;71 (1):65-72.

[151] Bukrinsky MI, Nottet HS, Schmidtmayerova H, Dubrovsky L, Flanagan CR, Mullins ME, et al. Regulation of nitric oxide synthase activity in human immunodeficiency virus type 1 (HIV-1)-infected monocytes: implications for HIV-associated neurological disease. J Exp Med. 1995 Feb 1;181 (2):735-45.

[152] Piette J, Legrand-Poels S. HIV-1 reactivation after an oxidative stress mediated by different reactive oxygen species. Chem Biol Interact. 1994 Jun;91 (2-3):79-89.

[153] Szydlowska K, Tymianski M. Calcium, ischemia and excitotoxicity. Cell Calcium. 2010 Feb;47 (2):122-9.

[154] Jiang ZG, Piggee C, Heyes MP, Murphy C, Quearry B, Bauer M, et al. Glutamate is a mediator of neurotoxicity in secretions of activated HIV-1-infected macrophages. Journal of neuroimmunology. 2001 Jul 2;117 (1-2):97-107.

[155] Erdmann N, Zhao J, Lopez AL, Herek S, Curthoys N, Hexum TD, et al. Glutamate production by HIV-1 infected human macrophage is blocked by the inhibition of glutaminase. J Neurochem. 2007 Jul;102 (2):539-49.

[156] Zhao J, Lopez AL, Erichsen D, Herek S, Cotter RL, Curthoys NP, et al. Mitochondrial glutaminase enhances extracellular glutamate production in HIV-1-infected macrophages: linkage to HIV-1 associated dementia. J Neurochem. 2004 Jan;88 (1):169-80.

[157] Huang Y, Zhao L, Jia B, Wu L, Li Y, Curthoys N, et al. Glutaminase dysregulation in HIV-1-infected human microglia mediates neurotoxicity: relevant to HIV-1-associated neurocognitive disorders. J Neurosci. 2011 Oct 19;31 (42):15195-204.

[158] Banerjee A, Zhang X, Manda KR, Banks WA, Ercal N. HIV proteins (gp120 and Tat) and methamphetamine in oxidative stress-induced damage in the brain: potential role of the thiol antioxidant N-acetylcysteine amide. Free Radic Biol Med. 2010 May 15;48 (10):1388-98.

[159] Price TO, Ercal N, Nakaoke R, Banks WA. HIV-1 viral proteins gp120 and Tat induce oxidative stress in brain endothelial cells. Brain Res. 2005 May 31;1045 (1-2):57-63.

[160] Viviani B, Corsini E, Binaglia M, Galli CL, Marinovich M. Reactive oxygen species generated by glia are responsible for neuron death induced by human immunodeficiency virus-glycoprotein 120 in vitro. Neuroscience. 2001;107 (1):51-8.

[161] Dawson VL, Dawson TM, Uhl GR, Snyder SH. Human immunodeficiency virus type 1 coat protein neurotoxicity mediated by nitric oxide in primary cortical cultures. Proc Natl Acad Sci U S A. 1993 Apr 15;90 (8):3256-9.

[162] Pietraforte D, Tritarelli E, Testa U, Minetti M. gp120 HIV envelope glycoprotein increases the production of nitric oxide in human monocyte-derived macrophages. J Leukoc Biol. 1994 Feb;55 (2):175-82.

[163] Kruman, II, Nath A, Mattson MP. HIV-1 protein Tat induces apoptosis of hippocampal neurons by a mechanism involving caspase activation, calcium overload, and oxidative stress. Exp Neurol. 1998 Dec;154 (2):276-88.

[164] Toborek M, Lee YW, Pu H, Malecki A, Flora G, Garrido R, et al. HIV-Tat protein induces oxidative and inflammatory pathways in brain endothelium. J Neurochem. 2003 Jan;84 (1):169-79.

[165] Israel N, Gougerot-Pocidalo MA. Oxidative stress in human immunodeficiency virus infection. Cell Mol Life Sci. 1997 Dec;53 (11-12):864-70.

[166] Flores SC, Marecki JC, Harper KP, Bose SK, Nelson SK, McCord JM. Tat protein of human immunodeficiency virus type 1 represses expression of manganese superoxide dismutase in HeLa cells. Proc Natl Acad Sci U S A. 1993 Aug 15;90 (16):7632-6.

[167] Aksenov MY, Hasselrot U, Bansal AK, Wu G, Nath A, Anderson C, et al. Oxidative damage induced by the injection of HIV-1 Tat protein in the rat striatum. Neurosci Lett. 2001 Jun 1;305 (1):5-8.

[168] Raidel SM, Haase C, Jansen NR, Russ RB, Sutliff RL, Velsor LW, et al. Targeted myocardial transgenic expression of HIV Tat causes cardiomyopathy and mitochondrial damage. Am J Physiol Heart Circ Physiol. 2002 May;282 (5):H1672-8.

[169] Choi J, Liu RM, Kundu RK, Sangiorgi F, Wu W, Maxson R, et al. Molecular mechanism of decreased glutathione content in human immunodeficiency virus type 1 Tat-transgenic mice. J Biol Chem. 2000 Feb 4;275 (5):3693-8.

[170] Westendorp MO, Shatrov VA, Schulze-Osthoff K, Frank R, Kraft M, Los M, et al. HIV-1 Tat potentiates TNF-induced NF-kappa B activation and cytotoxicity by altering the cellular redox state. The EMBO journal. 1995 Feb 1;14 (3):546-54.

[171] Deshmane SL, Mukerjee R, Fan S, Del Valle L, Michiels C, Sweet T, et al. Activation of the oxidative stress pathway by HIV-1 Vpr leads to induction of hypoxia-inducible factor 1alpha expression. J Biol Chem. 2009 Apr 24;284 (17):11364-73.

[172] Ferrucci A, Nonnemacher MR, Cohen EA, Wigdahl B. Extracellular human immunodeficiency virus type 1 viral protein R causes reductions in astrocytic ATP and glutathione levels compromising the antioxidant reservoir. Virus Res. 2012 Jun 9.

[173] Vidal F, Gutierrez F, Gutierrez M, Olona M, Sanchez V, Mateo G, et al. Pharmacoge-
       netics of adverse effects due to antiretroviral drugs. AIDS reviews. (Research Sup-
       port, Non-U.S. Gov'tReview). 2010 Jan-Mar;12 (1):15-30.

[174] Zhou H, Gurley EC, Jarujaron S, Ding H, Fang Y, Xu Z, Pandak WM, Hylemon PB.
       HIV protease inhibitors activate the unfolded protein response and disrupt lipid me-
       tabolism in primary hepatocytes. Am J Physiol Gastrointest Liver Physiol.
       2006;291:G1071-G80.

[175] Zhou H, Pandak WM, Lyall V, Natarajan R, Hylemon PB. HIV Protease Inhibitors
       Activate the Unfolded Protein Response in Macrophages: Implication for Atheroscle-
       rosis and Cardiovascular Disease. Mol Pharmacol. 2005;68:690-700.

[176] Letendre S, Marquie-Beck J, Capparelli E, Best B, Clifford D, Collier AC, et al. Valida-
       tion of the CNS Penetration-Effectiveness rank for quantifying antiretroviral penetra-
       tion into the central nervous system. Arch Neurol. 2008 Jan;65 (1):65-70.

[177] Letendre SL, Ellis RJ, Ances BM, McCutchan JA. Neurologic complications of HIV
       disease and their treatment. Top HIV Med. 2010 Apr-May;18 (2):45-55.

[178] Tozzi V, Balestra P, Salvatori MF, Vlassi C, Liuzzi G, Giancola ML, et al. Changes in
       Cognition During Antiretroviral Therapy: Comparison of 2 Different Ranking Sys-
       tems to Measure Antiretroviral Drug Efficacy on HIV-Associated Neurocognitive
       Disorders. JAIDS Journal of Acquired Immune Deficiency Syndromes. 2009;52 (1):
       56-63 10.1097/QAI.0b013e3181af83d6.

[179] Garvey L, Winston A, Walsh J, Post F, Porter K, Gazzard B, et al. Antiretroviral thera-
       py CNS penetration and HIV-1-associated CNS disease. Neurology. 2011 Feb 22;76
       (8):693-700.

[180] Lanoy E, Guiguet M, Bentata M, Rouveix E, Dhiver C, Poizot-Martin I, et al. Survival
       after neuroAIDS. Neurology. 2011 February 15, 2011;76 (7):644-51.

[181] Marra CM, Zhao Y, Clifford DB, Letendre S, Evans S, Henry K, et al. Impact of com-
       bination antiretroviral therapy on cerebrospinal fluid HIV RNA and neurocognitive
       performance. AIDS (London, England). 2009 Jul 17;23 (11):1359-66.

[182] Smurzynski M, Wu K, Letendre S, Robertson K, Bosch RJ, Clifford DB, et al. Effects
       of central nervous system antiretroviral penetration on cognitive functioning in the
       ALLRT cohort. AIDS (London, England). 2011;25 (3):357-65 10.1097/QAD.
       0b013e32834171f8.

[183] Cysique LA, Vaida F, Letendre S, Gibson S, Cherner M, Woods SP, et al. Dynamics of
       cognitive change in impaired HIV-positive patients initiating antiretroviral therapy.
       Neurology. 2009 August 4, 2009;73 (5):342-8.

[184] Marra CM, Zhao Y, Clifford DB, Letendre S, Evans S, Henry K, et al. Impact of com-
       bination antiretroviral therapy on cerebrospinal fluid HIV RNA and neurocognitive
       performance. AIDS. 2009 Jul 17;23(11):1359-66.

[185]   Ramirez SH, Potula R, Fan S, Eidem T, Papugani A, Reichenbach N, et al. Metham-
        phetamine disrupts blood-brain barrier function by induction of oxidative stress in
        brain endothelial cells. J Cereb Blood Flow Metab. 2009 Dec;29 (12):1933-45.

[186]   Shiu C, Barbier E, Di Cello F, Choi HJ, Stins M. HIV-1 gp120 as well as alcohol affect
        blood-brain barrier permeability and stress fiber formation: involvement of reactive
        oxygen species. Alcohol Clin Exp Res. 2007 Jan;31 (1):130-7.

[187]   Qin L, He J, Hanes RN, Pluzarev O, Hong JS, Crews FT. Increased systemic and brain
        cytokine production and neuroinflammation by endotoxin following ethanol treat-
        ment. J Neuroinflammation. 2008;5:10.

[188]   Ferraresi R, Troiano L, Roat E, Nemes E, Lugli E, Nasi M, et al. Protective effect of
        acetyl-L-carnitine against oxidative stress induced by antiretroviral drugs. FEBS let-
        ters. 2006 Dec 11;580 (28-29):6612-6.

[189]   Manda K, Banerjee A, Banks WA, Ercal N. Highly active antiretroviral therapy drug
        combination induces oxidative stress and mitochondrial dysfunction in immortalized
        human blood-brain barrier endothelial cells. Free Rad Biol and Med. 2011;50:801-10.

[190]   Brandmann M, Tulpule K, Schmidt MM, Dringen R. The antiretroviral protease in-
        hibitors indinavir and nelfinavir stimulate Mrp1-mediated GSH export from cultured
        brain astrocytes. J Neurochem. 2012 Jan;120 (1):78-92.

[191]   Touzet O, Philips A. Resveratrol protects against protease inhibitor-induced reactive
        oxygen species production, reticulum stress and lipid raft perturbation. AIDS (Lon-
        don, England). 2010 Jun 19, 2010;24 (10):1437-47.

[192]   Lewis W, Gonzalez B, Chomyn A, Papoian T. Zidovudine induces molecular, bio-
        chemical, and ultrastructural changes in rat skeletal muscle mitochondria. J Clin In-
        vest. 1992 Apr;89 (4):1354-60.

[193]   Gao RY, Mukhopadhyay P, Mohanraj R, Wang H, Horvath B, Yin S, et al. Resveratrol
        attenuates azidothymidine-induced cardiotoxicity by decreasing mitochondrial reac-
        tive oxygen species generation in human cardiomyocytes. Mol Med Report. 2011 Jan-
        Feb;4 (1):151-5.

[194]   de la Asuncion JG, del Olmo ML, Sastre J, Pallardo FV, Vina J. Zidovudine (AZT)
        causes an oxidation of mitochondrial DNA in mouse liver. Hepatology. 1999 Mar;29
        (3):985-7.

[195]   de la Asuncion JG, Del Olmo ML, Gomez-Cambronero LG, Sastre J, Pallardo FV, Vi-
        na J. AZT induces oxidative damage to cardiac mitochondria: protective effect of vi-
        tamins C and E. Life Sci. 2004 Nov 19;76 (1):47-56.

[196]   Bialkowska A, Bialkowski K, Gerschenson M, Diwan BA, Jones AB, Olivero OA, et
        al. Oxidative DNA damage in fetal tissues after transplacental exposure to 3'-azi-
        do-3'-deoxythymidine (AZT). Carcinogenesis. 2000 May;21 (5):1059-62.

[197] Yamaguchi T, Katoh I, Kurata S. Azidothymidine causes functional and structural destruction of mitochondria, glutathione deficiency and HIV-1 promoter sensitization. Eur J Biochem. 2002 Jun;269 (11):2782-8.

[198] Velsor LW, Kovacevic M, Goldstein M, Leitner HM, Lewis W, Day BJ. Mitochondrial oxidative stress in human hepatoma cells exposed to stavudine. Toxicol Appl Pharmacol. 2004 Aug 15;199 (1):10-9.

[199] Gerschenson M, Nguyen VT, St Claire MC, Harbaugh SW, Harbaugh JW, Proia LA, et al. Chronic stavudine exposure induces hepatic mitochondrial toxicity in adult Erythrocebus patas monkeys. J Hum Virol. 2001 Nov-Dec;4 (6):335-42.

[200] Opii WO, Sultana R, Abdul HM, Ansari MA, Nath A, Butterfield DA. Oxidative stress and toxicity induced by the nucleoside reverse transcriptase inhibitor (NRTI)--2',3'-dideoxycytidine (ddC): relevance to HIV-dementia. Exp Neurol. 2007 Mar;204 (1):29-38.

[201] Apostolova N, Gomez-Sucerquia LJ, Moran A, Alvarez A, Blas-Garcia A, Esplugues JV. Enhanced oxidative stress and increased mitochondrial mass during efavirenz-induced apoptosis in human hepatic cells. Br J Pharmacol. 2010 Aug;160 (8):2069-84.

[202] Ciccarelli N, Fabbiani M, Di Giambenedetto S, Fanti I, Baldonero E, Bracciale L, et al. Efavirenz associated with cognitive disorders in otherwise asymptomatic HIV-infected patients. Neurology. 2011 Apr 19;76 (16):1403-9.

[203] Chai H, Yan S, Lin P, Lumsden AB, Yao Q, Chen C. Curcumin blocks HIV protease inhibitor ritonavir-induced vascular dysfunction in porcine coronary arteries. J Am Coll Surg. 2005 Jun;200 (6):820-30.

[204] Vincent S, Tourniaire F, El Yazidi CM, Compe E, Manches O, Plannels R, et al. Nelfinavir induces necrosis of 3T3F44-2A adipocytes by oxidative stress. Journal of acquired immune deficiency syndromes (1999). 2004 Dec 15;37 (5):1556-62.

[205] Amatore C, Arbault S, Jaouen G, Koh AC, Leong WK, Top S, et al. Pro-oxidant properties of AZT and other thymidine analogues in macrophages: implication of the azido moiety in oxidative stress. ChemMedChem. 2010 Feb 1;5 (2):296-301.

[206] Jensen BK, Akay C, Lindl KA, Jordan-Sciutto K. Involvement of the Antioxidant response pathway in neuroglial, neuronal, and astrocytic cultures exposed to antiretroviral compounds.. The International Symposium on NeuroVirology; New York, NY, USA. Journal of NeuroVirology2012. p. S51.

[207] Akay C, Cooper M, Odeleye A, Jensen BK, White M, Vassoler F, et al. Antiretroviral Drugs Induce Oxidative Stress and Neuronal Damage in the Central Nervous System. The International Symposium on NeuroVirology; 2012; New York, N.Y., USA: Journal of NeuroVirology; 2012. p. S5.

[208] Li W, Kong A. Molecular Mechanisms of Nrf2-Mediated Antioxidant Response. Molecular Carcinogenesis. 2009;48:91-104.

[209] Shih A, Johnson DA, Wong G, Kraft AD, Jiang L, Erb H, Johnson JA, Murphy TH. Coordinate Regulation of Glutathione Biosynthesis and Release by Nrf2-Expressing Glia Potently Protects Neurons from Oxidative Stress. J Neurosci. 2003;23 (8): 3394-406.

[210] Cross SA, Cook DR, Chi AW, Vance PJ, Kolson LL, Wong BJ, et al. Dimethyl fumarate, an immune modulator and inducer of the antioxidant response, suppresses HIV replication and macrophage-mediated neurotoxicity: a novel candidate for HIV neuroprotection. J Immunol. (Research Support, N.I.H., Extramural). 2011 Nov 15;187 (10):5015-25.

[211] Weakley SM, Jiang J, Lu J, Wang X, Lin PH, Yao Q, et al. Natural antioxidant dihydroxybenzyl alcohol blocks ritonavir-induced endothelial dysfunction in porcine pulmonary arteries and human endothelial cells. Med Sci Monit. 2011 Sep;17 (9):BR235-41.

[212] Meulendyke KA, Pletnikov MV, Engle EL, Tarwater PM, Graham DR, Zink MC. Early minocycline treatment prevents a decrease in striatal dopamine in an SIV model of HIV-associated neurological disease. J Neuroimmune Pharmacol. 2012 Jun;7 (2): 454-64.

[213] Jariwalla RJ, Lalezari J, Cenko D, Mansour SE, Kumar A, Gangapurkar B, et al. Restoration of blood total glutathione status and lymphocyte function following alpha-lipoic acid supplementation in patients with HIV infection. J Altern Complement Med. 2008 Mar;14 (2):139-46.

[214] Batterham M, Gold J, Naidoo D, Lux O, Sadler S, Bridle S, et al. A preliminary open label dose comparison using an antioxidant regimen to determine the effect on viral load and oxidative stress in men with HIV/AIDS. Eur J Clin Nutr. 2001 Feb;55 (2): 107-14.

[215] Kutzing MK, Luo V, Firestein BL. Protection from glutamate-induced excitotoxicity by memantine. Ann Biomed Eng. 2012 May;40 (5):1170-81.

[216] Nagatsu T, Sawada M. Molecular mechanism of the relation of monoamine oxidase B and its inhibitors to Parkinson's disease: possible implications of glial cells. J Neural Transm Suppl. 2006 (71):53-65.

[217] Schifitto G, Yiannoutsos CT, Ernst T, Navia BA, Nath A, Sacktor N, et al. Selegiline and oxidative stress in HIV-associated cognitive impairment. Neurology. 2009 Dec 8;73 (23):1975-81.

[218] Bhaskaran K, Mussini C, Antinori A, Walker AS, Dorrucci M, Sabin C, et al. Changes in the incidence and predictors of human immunodeficiency virus-associated dementia in the era of highly active antiretroviral therapy. Ann Neurol. 2008 Feb;63 (2): 213-21.

[219] Nath A. Human immunodeficiency virus-associated neurocognitive disorder: pathophysiology in relation to drug addiction. Ann N Y Acad Sci. 2010 Feb;1187:122-8.

[220] Cadet J, Krasnova I. Interactions of HIV and methamphetamine: Cellular and molecular mechanisms of toxicity potentiation. Neurotoxicity Research. 2007;12 (3):181-204.

[221] Durazzo TC, Rothlind JC, Cardenas VA, Studholme C, Weiner MW, Meyerhoff DJ. Chronic cigarette smoking and heavy drinking in human immunodeficiency virus: consequences for neurocognition and brain morphology. Alcohol. 2007 Nov;41 (7): 489-501.

[222] Miguez-Burbano MJ, Lewis JE, Moreno J, Fishman J. Cognitive performance and the thymus among HIV-infected subjects receiving HAART. Biologics. 2008 Jun;2 (2): 321-7.

[223] Miguez-Burbano MJ, Nair M, Lewis JE, Fishman J. The role of alcohol on platelets, thymus and cognitive performance among HIV-infected subjects: are they related? Platelets. 2009 Jun;20 (4):260-7.

[224] Winston A, Garvey L, Scotney E, Yerrakalva D, Allsop JM, Thomson EC, et al. Does acute hepatitis C infection affect the central nervous system in HIV-1 infected individuals? J Viral Hepat. 2010 Jun;17 (6):419-26.

[225] Malaspina L, Woods SP, Moore DJ, Depp C, Letendre SL, Jeste D, et al. Successful cognitive aging in persons living with HIV infection. J Neurovirol. Feb;17 (1):110-9.

[226] Mateen FJ, Mills EJ. Aging and HIV-related cognitive loss. Jama. Jul 25;308 (4):349-50.

[227] Deeks SG. Immune dysfunction, inflammation, and accelerated aging in patients on antiretroviral therapy. Top HIV Med. 2009 Sep-Oct;17 (4):118-23.

[228] Xu J, Ikezu T. The comorbidity of HIV-associated neurocognitive disorders and Alzheimer's disease: a foreseeable medical challenge in post-HAART era. J Neuroimmune Pharmacol. 2009 Jun;4 (2):200-12.

[229] Tisch S, Brew B. Parkinsonism in hiv-infected patients on highly active antiretroviral therapy. Neurology. 2009 Aug 4;73 (5):401-3.

[230] Alisky JM. The coming problem of HIV-associated Alzheimer's disease. Medical hypotheses. 2007;69 (5):1140-3.

[231] Holt JL, Kraft-Terry SD, Chang L. Neuroimaging studies of the aging HIV-1-infected brain. J Neurovirol. Aug;18 (4):291-302.

[232] Gannon P, Khan MZ, Kolson DL. Current understanding of HIV-associated neurocognitive disorders pathogenesis. Curr Opin Neurol. Jun;24 (3):275-83.

[233] Anthony ICB, J.E. Neuropathological Findings Associated with Long-Term HAART. In: Paul RS, NC; Valcour, V; Tasima, KT, editor. HIV and the Brain: New Challenges in the Modern Era: Humana Press; 2009. p. 1-19.

[234] Brew BJ, Crowe SM, Landay A, Cysique LA, Guillemin G. Neurodegeneration and ageing in the HAART era. J Neuroimmune Pharmacol. 2009 Jun;4 (2):163-74.

[235] Sacktor N, Lyles RH, Skolasky R, Kleeberger C, Selnes OA, Miller EN, et al. HIV-associated neurologic disease incidence changes:: Multicenter AIDS Cohort Study, 1990-1998. Neurology. 2001 Jan 23;56 (2):257-60.

[236] Martin CP, Fain MJ, Klotz SA. The older HIV-positive adult: a critical review of the medical literature. Am J Med. 2008 Dec;121 (12):1032-7.

[237] Kalayjian RC, Landay A, Pollard RB, Taub DD, Gross BH, Francis IR, et al. Age-related immune dysfunction in health and in human immunodeficiency virus (HIV) disease: association of age and HIV infection with naive CD8+ cell depletion, reduced expression of CD28 on CD8+ cells, and reduced thymic volumes. J Infect Dis. 2003 Jun 15;187 (12):1924-33.

[238] Kirk JB, Goetz MB. Human immunodeficiency virus in an aging population, a complication of success. Journal of the American Geriatrics Society. 2009 Nov;57 (11): 2129-38.

[239] Butt AA, Dascomb KK, DeSalvo KB, Bazzano L, Kissinger PJ, Szerlip HM. Human immunodeficiency virus infection in elderly patients. Southern medical journal. 2001 Apr;94 (4):397-400.

[240] Manfredi R. HIV disease and advanced age: an increasing therapeutic challenge. Drugs & aging. 2002;19 (9):647-69.

[241] Goetz MB, Boscardin WJ, Wiley D, Alkasspooles S. Decreased recovery of CD4 lymphocytes in older HIV-infected patients beginning highly active antiretroviral therapy. AIDS (London, England). 2001 Aug 17;15 (12):1576-9.

[242] Thompson MA, Aberg JA, Cahn P, Montaner JS, Rizzardini G, Telenti A, et al. Antiretroviral treatment of adult HIV infection: 2010 recommendations of the International AIDS Society-USA panel. Jama. Jul 21;304 (3):321-33.

[243] Spengler U. Management of end-stage liver disease in HIV/hepatitis C virus co-infection. Curr Opin HIV AIDS. Nov;6 (6):527-33.

[244] Desquilbet L, Jacobson LP, Fried LP, Phair JP, Jamieson BD, Holloway M, et al. HIV-1 infection is associated with an earlier occurrence of a phenotype related to frailty. The journals of gerontology. 2007 Nov;62 (11):1279-86.

[245] Patel P, Hanson DL, Sullivan PS, Novak RM, Moorman AC, Tong TC, et al. Incidence of types of cancer among HIV-infected persons compared with the general population in the United States, 1992-2003. Ann Intern Med. 2008 May 20;148 (10):728-36.

[246] Zhou H, Pandak WM, Jr., Lyall V, Natarajan R, Hylemon PB. HIV protease inhibitors activate the unfolded protein response in macrophages: implication for atherosclerosis and cardiovascular disease. Molecular pharmacology. 2005 Sep;68 (3):690-700.

[247] Bozzette SA, Ake CF, Tam HK, Chang SW, Louis TA. Cardiovascular and cerebrovascular events in patients treated for human immunodeficiency virus infection. The New England journal of medicine. 2003 Feb 20;348 (8):702-10.

[248] Cherner M, Ellis RJ, Lazzaretto D, Young C, Mindt MR, Atkinson JH, et al. Effects of HIV-1 infection and aging on neurobehavioral functioning: preliminary findings. AIDS (London, England). 2004 Jan 1;18 Suppl 1:S27-34.

[249] Sacktor N, Skolasky R, Selnes OA, Watters M, Poff P, Shiramizu B, et al. Neuropsychological test profile differences between young and old human immunodeficiency virus-positive individuals. J Neurovirol. 2007 Jun;13 (3):203-9.

[250] Chang L, Yakupov R, Nakama H, Stokes B, Ernst T. Antiretroviral treatment is associated with increased attentional load-dependent brain activation in HIV patients. J Neuroimmune Pharmacol. 2008 Jun;3 (2):95-104.

[251] Gongvatana A, Cohen RA, Correia S, Devlin KN, Miles J, Kang H, et al. Clinical contributors to cerebral white matter integrity in HIV-infected individuals. J Neurovirol. Oct;17 (5):477-86.

[252] Towgood KJ, Pitkanen M, Kulasegaram R, Fradera A, Kumar A, Soni S, et al. Mapping the brain in younger and older asymptomatic HIV-1 men: frontal volume changes in the absence of other cortical or diffusion tensor abnormalities. Cortex. Feb;48 (2):230-41.

[253] Ernst T, Chang L. Effect of aging on brain metabolism in antiretroviral-naive HIV patients. AIDS (London, England). 2004 Jan 1;18 Suppl 1:S61-7.

[254] Harezlak J, Buchthal S, Taylor M, Schifitto G, Zhong J, Daar E, et al. Persistence of HIV-associated cognitive impairment, inflammation, and neuronal injury in era of highly active antiretroviral treatment. AIDS (London, England). Mar 13;25 (5):625-33.

[255] Anthony IC, Ramage SN, Carnie FW, Simmonds P, Bell JE. Influence of HAART on HIV-related CNS disease and neuroinflammation. J Neuropathol Exp Neurol. 2005 Jun;64 (6):529-36.

[256] Brew BJ. Evidence for a change in AIDS dementia complex in the era of highly active antiretroviral therapy and the possibility of new forms of AIDS dementia complex. AIDS (London, England). 2004 Jan 1;18 Suppl 1:S75-8.

[257] Anthony IC, Ramage SN, Carnie FW, Simmonds P, Bell JE. Accelerated Tau deposition in the brains of individuals infected with human immunodeficiency virus-1 before and after the advent of highly active anti-retroviral therapy. Acta Neuropathol. 2006 Jun;111 (6):529-38.

[258] Ances BM, Benzinger TL, Christensen JJ, Thomas J, Venkat R, Teshome M, et al. 11C-PiB imaging of human immunodeficiency virus-associated neurocognitive disorder. Arch Neurol. Jan;69 (1):72-7.

[259] Green DA, Masliah E, Vinters HV, Beizai P, Moore DJ, Achim CL. Brain deposition of beta-amyloid is a common pathologic feature in HIV positive patients. AIDS (London, England). 2005 Mar 4;19 (4):407-11.

[260] Rempel HC, Pulliam L. HIV-1 Tat inhibits neprilysin and elevates amyloid beta. AIDS (London, England). 2005 Jan 28;19 (2):127-35.

[261] Brew BJ, Pemberton L, Blennow K, Wallin A, Hagberg L. CSF amyloid beta42 and tau levels correlate with AIDS dementia complex. Neurology. 2005 Nov 8;65 (9): 1490-2.

[262] Esiri MM, Biddolph SC, Morris CS. Prevalence of Alzheimer plaques in AIDS. J Neurol Neurosurg Psychiatry. 1998 Jul;65 (1):29-33.

[263] Cysique LA, Maruff P, Brew BJ. Prevalence and pattern of neuropsychological impairment in human immunodeficiency virus-infected/acquired immunodeficiency syndrome (HIV/AIDS) patients across pre- and post-highly active antiretroviral therapy eras: a combined study of two cohorts. J Neurovirol. 2004 Dec;10 (6):350-7.

[264] Cysique LA, Brew BJ. Neuropsychological functioning and antiretroviral treatment in HIV/AIDS: a review. Neuropsychol Rev. 2009 Jun;19 (2):169-85.

[265] Achim CL, Adame A, Dumaop W, Everall IP, Masliah E. Increased accumulation of intraneuronal amyloid beta in HIV-infected patients. J Neuroimmune Pharmacol. 2009 Jun;4 (2):190-9.

[266] Chen CH, Vazquez-Padua M, Cheng YC. Effect of anti-human immunodeficiency virus nucleoside analogs on mitochondrial DNA and its implication for delayed toxicity. Mol Pharmacol. 1991 May;39 (5):625-8.

[267] Dalakas MC. Peripheral neuropathy and antiretroviral drugs. J Peripher Nerv Syst. 2001 Mar;6 (1):14-20.

[268] Schweinsburg BC, Taylor MJ, Alhassoon OM, Gonzalez R, Brown GG, Ellis RJ, et al. Brain mitochondrial injury in human immunodeficiency virus-seropositive (HIV+) individuals taking nucleoside reverse transcriptase inhibitors. J Neurovirol. 2005 Aug;11 (4):356-64.

[269] Dufer M, Neye Y, Krippeit-Drews P, Drews G. Direct interference of HIV protease inhibitors with pancreatic beta-cell function. Naunyn Schmiedebergs Arch Pharmacol. 2004 Jun;369 (6):583-90.

[270] Zhou H, Gurley EC, Jarujaron S, Ding H, Fang Y, Xu Z, et al. HIV protease inhibitors activate the unfolded protein response and disrupt lipid metabolism in primary hepatocytes. American journal of physiology. 2006 Dec;291 (6):G1071-80.

[271] Schutt M, Zhou J, Meier M, Klein HH. Long-term effects of HIV-1 protease inhibitors on insulin secretion and insulin signaling in INS-1 beta cells. J Endocrinol. 2004 Dec; 183 (3):445-54.

[272] Liang JS, Distler O, Cooper DA, Jamil H, Deckelbaum RJ, Ginsberg HN, et al. HIV protease inhibitors protect apolipoprotein B from degradation by the proteasome: a potential mechanism for protease inhibitor-induced hyperlipidemia. Nat Med. 2001 Dec;7 (12):1327-31.

[273] Schubert M, Gautam D, Surjo D, Ueki K, Baudler S, Schubert D, et al. Role for neuronal insulin resistance in neurodegenerative diseases. Proc Natl Acad Sci U S A. 2004
Mar 2;101 (9):3100-5.

[274] Steen E, Terry BM, Rivera EJ, Cannon JL, Neely TR, Tavares R, et al. Impaired insulin
and insulin-like growth factor expression and signaling mechanisms in Alzheimer's
disease--is this type 3 diabetes? J Alzheimers Dis. 2005 Feb;7 (1):63-80.

[275] Kroner Z. The relationship between Alzheimer's disease and diabetes: Type 3 diabetes? Altern Med Rev. 2009 Dec;14 (4):373-9.

[276] Moyle G. Mechanisms of HIV and nucleoside reverse transcriptase inhibitor injury to
mitochondria. Antivir Ther. 2005;10 Suppl 2:M47-52.

[277] Robertson KR, Smurzynski M, Parsons TD, Wu K, Bosch RJ, Wu J, et al. The prevalence and incidence of neurocognitive impairment in the HAART era. AIDS (London,
England). 2007 Sep 12;21 (14):1915-21.

[278] Cook-Easterwood J, Middaugh LD, Griffin WC, 3rd, Khan I, Tyor WR. Highly active
antiretroviral therapy of cognitive dysfunction and neuronal abnormalities in SCID
mice with HIV encephalitis. Exp Neurol. 2007 Jun;205 (2):506-12.

[279] Heaton RK, Clifford DB, Franklin DR, Jr., Woods SP, Ake C, Vaida F, et al. HIV-associated neurocognitive disorders persist in the era of potent antiretroviral therapy:
CHARTER Study. Neurology. 2010;75 (23):2087-96.

[280] Joska JA, Gouse H, Paul RH, Stein DJ, Flisher AJ. Does highly active antiretroviral
therapy improve neurocognitive function? A systematic review. J Neurovirol. Mar;16
(2):101-14.

[281] Smurzynski M, Wu K, Letendre S, Robertson K, Bosch RJ, Clifford DB, et al. Effects
of central nervous system antiretroviral penetration on cognitive functioning in the
ALLRT cohort. AIDS (London, England). Jan 28;25 (3):357-65.

[282] Letendre SL, McCutchan JA, Childers ME, Woods SP, Lazzaretto D, Heaton RK, et al.
Enhancing antiretroviral therapy for human immunodeficiency virus cognitive disorders. Ann Neurol. 2004 Sep;56 (3):416-23.

[283] Winston A, Duncombe C, Li PC, Gill JM, Kerr SJ, Puls R, et al. Does choice of combination antiretroviral therapy (cART) alter changes in cerebral function testing after
48 weeks in treatment-naive, HIV-1-infected individuals commencing cART? A
randomized, controlled study. Clin Infect Dis. Mar 15;50 (6):920-9.

Permissions

The contributors of this book come from diverse backgrounds, making this book a truly international effort. This book will bring forth new frontiers with its revolutionizing research information and detailed analysis of the nascent developments around the world.

We would like to thank Shailendra K. Saxena, PhD, DCAP, FAEB, for lending his expertise to make the book truly unique. He has played a crucial role in the development of this book. Without his invaluable contribution this book wouldn't have been possible. He has made vital efforts to compile up to date information on the varied aspects of this subject to make this book a valuable addition to the collection of many professionals and students.

This book was conceptualized with the vision of imparting up-to-date information and advanced data in this field. To ensure the same, a matchless editorial board was set up. Every individual on the board went through rigorous rounds of assessment to prove their worth. After which they invested a large part of their time researching and compiling the most relevant data for our readers. Conferences and sessions were held from time to time between the editorial board and the contributing authors to present the data in the most comprehensible form. The editorial team has worked tirelessly to provide valuable and valid information to help people across the globe.

Every chapter published in this book has been scrutinized by our experts. Their significance has been extensively debated. The topics covered herein carry significant findings which will fuel the growth of the discipline. They may even be implemented as practical applications or may be referred to as a beginning point for another development. Chapters in this book were first published by InTech; hereby published with permission under the Creative Commons Attribution License or equivalent.

The editorial board has been involved in producing this book since its inception. They have spent rigorous hours researching and exploring the diverse topics which have resulted in the successful publishing of this book. They have passed on their knowledge of decades through this book. To expedite this challenging task, the publisher supported the team at every step. A small team of assistant editors was also appointed to further simplify the editing procedure and attain best results for the readers.

Our editorial team has been hand-picked from every corner of the world. Their multi-ethnicity adds dynamic inputs to the discussions which result in innovative outcomes. These outcomes are then further discussed with the researchers and contributors who give their valuable feedback and opinion regarding the same. The feedback is then collaborated with the researches and they are edited in a comprehensive manner to aid the understanding of the subject.

Apart from the editorial board, the designing team has also invested a significant amount of their time in understanding the subject and creating the most relevant covers. They scrutinized every image to scout for the most suitable representation of the subject and create an appropriate cover for the book.

The publishing team has been involved in this book since its early stages. They were actively engaged in every process, be it collecting the data, connecting with the contributors or procuring relevant information. The team has been an ardent support to the editorial, designing and production team. Their endless efforts to recruit the best for this project, has resulted in the accomplishment of this book. They are a veteran in the field of academics and their pool of knowledge is as vast as their experience in printing. Their expertise and guidance has proved useful at every step. Their uncompromising quality standards have made this book an exceptional effort. Their encouragement from time to time has been an inspiration for everyone.

The publisher and the editorial board hope that this book will prove to be a valuable piece of knowledge for researchers, students, practitioners and scholars across the globe.

List of Contributors

Wilfried Posch, Cornelia Lass-Flörl and Doris Wilflingseder
Innsbruck Medical University, Division of Hygiene and Medical Microbiology, Innsbruck, Austria

Abdulkarim Alhetheel
Department of Microbiology, Faculty of Medicine, King Saud University, Riyadh, Saudi Arabia

Mahmoud Aly
King Abdullah International Medical Research Center, National Guard Hospital, Riyadh, Saudi Arabia

Marko Kryworuchko
Department of Veterinary Microbiology, Western College of Veterinary Medicine, University of Saskatchewan, Saskatoon, Canada

Nitya Nathwani
City of Hope National Medical Center, Duarte, USA

Chi Dola, Maga Martinez, Olivia Chang and Amanda Johnson
Department of Obstetrics and Gynecology, Tulane University School of Medicine, New Orleans, Louisiana, USA

Teddy Charles Adias
Bayelsa State College of Health Technology, Ogbia Town, Yenagoa, Nigeria

Osaro Erhabor
Department of Blood Sciences, Royal Bolton Hospital NHS Trust UK, Bolton, United Kingdom

Shailendra K. Saxena and Sneham Tiwari
Centre for Cellular and Molecular Biology (CCMB-CSIR), Hyderabad, India

Madhavan P.N. Nair
College of Medicine, Florida International University, Miami, USA

Rehana Basri and Wan Mohamad Wan Majdiah
Neurology Craniofacial Sciences & Oral Biology, School of Dental Science, Universiti Sains, Malaysia

Peter J. Chipimo
University of Bergen, Faculty of Medicine, Centre for International Health, Norway University of Zambia, School of Medicine, Department of Public Health, Zambia

Knut Fylkesnes
University of Bergen, Faculty of Medicine, Centre for International Health, Norway

Jennifer M. King, Brigid K. Jensen, Patrick J. Gannon and Cagla Akay
Department of Pathology, School of Dental Medicine, University of Pennsylvania, Philadelphia, USA